HIV/AIDS Care and Treatment for People Who Inject Drugs in Asia and the Pacific

AN ESSENTIAL PRACTICE GUIDE

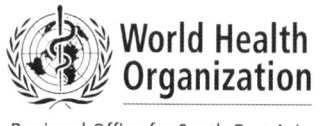
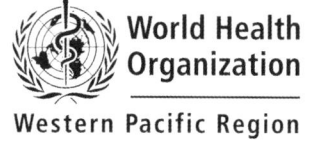
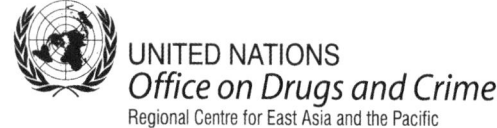

WHO Library Cataloguing in Publication Data

HIV/AIDS care and treatment for people who inject drugs in Asia and the Pacific: an essential practice guide.

1. HIV infections — prevention and control. 2. HIV infections — therapy.
3. Substance abuse, Intravenous. 4. Asia, Southeastern. Oceania. 6. Guidelines.

ISBN 978 92 9061 320 6   (NLM Classification: WC 503.2)

© World Health Organization 2008

All rights reserved.

The designations employed and the presentation of the material in this publication do not imply the expression of any opinion whatsoever on the part of the World Health Organization concerning the legal status of any country, territory, city or area, or of its authorities, or concerning the delimitation of its frontiers or boundaries. Dotted lines on maps represent approximate border lines for which there may not yet be full agreement.

The mention of specific companies or of certain manufacturers' products does not imply that they are endorsed or recommended by the World Health Organization in preference to others of a similar nature that are not mentioned. Errors and omissions excepted, the names of proprietary products are distinguished by initial capital letters.

The World Health Organization does not warrant that the information contained in this publication is complete and correct and shall not be liable for any damages incurred as a result of its use.

Publications of the World Health Organization can be obtained from WHO Press, World Health Organization, 20 Avenue Appia, 1211 Geneva 27, Switzerland (tel: +41 22 791 2476; fax: +41 22 791 4857; e-mail: bookorders@who.int). Requests for permission to reproduce WHO publications, in part or in whole, or to translate them – whether for sale or for noncommercial distribution – should be addressed to Publications, at the above address (fax: +41 22 791 4806; e-mail: permissions@who.int). For WHO Western Pacific Regional Publications, request for permission to reproduce should be addressed to Publications Office, World Health Organization, Regional Office for the Western Pacific, P.O. Box 2932, 1000, Manila, Philippines, fax: +63 2 521 1036, e-mail: publications@wpro.who.int

Table of Contents

Acknowledgements v
Abbreviations vii
Principles ix
Development of this treatment and care guide xi
Who is this guide for? xi

I. Background and general considerations 1
   1. Epidemiology of HIV and injecting drug use 1
   2. Health and social consequences of injecting drug use 2
      2.1. Health problems 2
      2.2. Social problems 3
         2.2.1. Stigma, discrimination and social marginalization 3
         2.2.2. Closed settings including prisons 4

II. Organization and management considerations 5
   1. Services for people who inject drugs 5
      1.1. General medical care 5
      1.2. Harm reduction 6
         1.2.1. Harm reduction programmes 8
      1.3. Drug dependence treatment and opioid substitution therapy 8
      1.4. Psychosocial support 9
   2. Models of comprehensive HIV/AIDS care for people who
      inject drugs 10
   3. Care within closed settings 10

III. Clinical management of HIV-infected people who inject drugs 12
   1. Initial patient evaluation 12
      1.1. Screening and assessment for substance dependence 12
         1.1.1. Screening 12
         1.1.2. Assessment 13
      1.2. Initial evaluation of a patient's HIV/AIDS status 13
      1.3. Psychosocial assessment 14
   2. Managing opioid dependence 15
      2.1. Opioid substitution therapies 16
         2.1.1. Methadone 16
         2.1.2. Buprenorphine 16
      2.2. Retention in treatment 17
      2.3. Multidisciplinary approach 17
      2.4. Detoxification programmes 18

3. Managing non-opioid dependence (including cocaine and ATS) 20
　　3.1. Symptoms experienced and medications used 20
　　3.2. Other interventions 21
4. Monitoring and evaluating effectiveness 21
5. Managing ART in HIV-infected people who inject drugs 21
　　5.1. Choice of ART regimen 24
6. Management of side-effects and toxicity 27
　　6.1. Immune reconstitution inflammatory syndrome (IRIS) 30
　　6.2. Hepatotoxicity of antiretroviral (ARV) drugs 31
7. Drug interactions with ARVs 31
　　7.1. Substitution medications 31
　　　　7.1.1. Methadone and ARVs 31
　　　　　　7.1.1.1. Mechanism of interactions between
　　　　　　　　　　methadone and ARVs 31
　　　　　　7.1.1.2. Management of the interactions between
　　　　　　　　　　other drugs, methadone and ARVs 31
　　　　7.1.2. Buprenorphine and ARVs 34
　　7.2. Interactions with illicit or recreational drugs 34
8. Adherence 35
　　8.1. Factors influencing adherence 36
　　8.2. Adherence support 36
　　　　8.2.1. Patient counselling 37
　　　　8.2.2. Other strategies 37
9. Management principles of acute and chronic pain relief
　　(including for people on OST) 38
10. Coinfections and comorbidities with HIV in people who
　　inject drugs 39
　　10.1. Hepatitis B (HBV) 39
　　10.2. Hepatitis C (HCV) 39
　　10.3. Chronic liver disease 39
　　10.4. Active tuberculosis (TB) and HIV/TB in people who
　　　　inject drugs 39
　　10.5. Other coinfections and comorbidities 41
　　10.6. Prevention of and support for treatment of coinfections
　　　　and comorbidities 41

References 42

Acknowledgements

This biregional guide for South-East Asia and the Western Pacific Regions is based on an early draft of the WHO European treatment protocols for injecting drug users and was adapted to the biregional context by Dr Mark Tyndall, University of British Columbia, BC Centre for Excellence in HIV/AIDS, Vancouver, Canada. Final revision before publication was done by Dr David Jacka (WPRO – Viet Nam) and Dr Marco Antônio de Àvila Vitória (WHO–HQ).

Many people have contributed to the development of this guide. The World Health Organization (WHO) wishes to thank all participants of the workshop "Developing treatment guidelines for injecting drug users" in Kuala Lumpur, Malaysia, May 2006 for their contribution.

WHO would particularly like to acknowledge the contribution of the technical advisory group who reviewed and revised these guidelines: Dr Dominique Ricard; Dr Emanuele Pontali; Dr Fábio Mesquita; Hathaikant (Boum) Ranumas; Dr Nguyen Tien Lam; Dr Rachel Burdon; and Umesh Sharma.

The publication was edited by Ms Manuela Moeller and Dr Fábio Mesquita (WPRO), Dr Ying-Ru Lo and Dr Mukta Sharma (SEARO), and Mr Gray Sattler (UNODC Regional Office in Bangkok). Technical editing was done by Dr Bandana Malhotra.

WHO acknowledges the generous contribution of the Canadian International Development Agency (CIDA) to the development of this publication.

WHO also acknowledges the partnership with UNODC in the final development of this publication.

ABBREVIATIONS

ABC	abacavir
AIDS	acquired immunodeficiency syndrome
APV	amprenavir
ARV	antiretroviral
ART	antiretroviral therapy
ATS	amphetamine-type stimulants
ASI	Addiction Severity Index
AUC	area under the curve
AZT	zidovudine (also known as ZDV)
BBV-TRAQ	Bloodborne virus transmission risk assessment questionnaire
CBT	cognitive–behavioural therapy
CMV	cytomegalovirus
CYP 450	cytochrome P450
ddI	didanosine
d4T	stavudine
DAART	directly administered antiretroviral therapy
DOT	directly observed therapy
DVT	deep venous thrombosis
EC	enteric coated
EFV	efavirenz
ELISA	enzyme-linked immunosorbent assay
FDC	fixed-dose combination
FTC	emtricitabine
GHB	gamma-hydroxybutyrate
Hb	haemoglobin
HBV	hepatitis B virus
HCV	hepatitis C virus
ICD-10	International Classification of Disease, 10th revision
IDU	injecting drug use
IDV	indinavir
IRIS	immune reconstitution inflammatory syndrome
HIV	human immunodeficiency virus
INH	isoniazid
LPV	lopinavir
MAC	*Mycobacterium avium* complex
MDMA	methylenedioxymethamphetamine
MDR	multidrug resistance
MSM	men who have sex with men
MTCT	mother-to-child transmission
NFV	nelfinavir
NGO	nongovernmental organization
NNRTI	non-nucleoside reverse transcriptase inhibitor
NRTI	nucleoside reverse transcriptase inhibitor
NVP	nevirapine

OI	opportunistic infection
OST	opioid substitution therapy
PCP	*Pneumocystis jiroveci* pneumonia (earlier known as *Pneumocystis carinii*)
PI	protease inhibitor
PLWHA	people living with HIV and AIDS
PMTCT	prevention of mother-to-child transmission
RNA	ribonucleic acid
RTV	ritonavir
SQV	saquinavir
SSRI	selective serotonin reuptake inhibitor
STI	sexually transmitted infection
THC	tetrahydrocannabinol
TLC	total lymphocyte count
TB	tuberculosis
TDF	tenofovir disoproxil fumarate
UNAIDS	United Nations Programme on HIV/AIDS
UNODC	United Nations Office on Drug and Crime
WBC	white blood cell (count)
WHO	World Health Organization
3TC	lamivudine

Principles

WHO, UNODC and others have committed to scaling up access to antiretroviral therapy (ART) and have confirmed that people who inject drugs should have equitable and universal access to HIV/AIDS prevention, care and treatment.[1] While this guide has been produced specifically for countries in the WHO South-East Asia and Western Pacific Regions, it will also be useful for countries where people who inject drugs are entering HIV/AIDS care and treatment.

While a large proportion of individuals with HIV in the South-East Asia and Western Pacific Regions inject drugs, they are much less likely to receive ART when compared with persons who have acquired HIV through other routes.[2-4] Globally, drug users have reduced access to and utilization of ART, and initiate treatment at more advanced stages of infection.[5] People with a history of injecting drug use (IDU) have lower rates of access to ART, even in developed countries with relatively good access in the general population.[6-9]

Studies show that some clinicians may be reluctant to prescribe ART to HIV-infected people who inject drugs, due to the common belief that such people have lower levels of adherence which, in turn, may lead to elevated rates of antiretroviral (ARV) resistance. Studies show that resistance to ARVs is similar among people who inject drugs and those who do not.[10] Where comprehensive HIV care has been provided to people who inject drugs in an accessible and non-judgemental way, high proportions of patients have been attracted to and retained in effective treatment. Combining HIV/AIDS care with substance dependence treatment services (including harm reduction, detoxification and opioid substitution therapy [OST]) and psychosocial services has been particularly successful.[11-13]

In addition to the general principles governing the care and treatment of people living with HIV/AIDS (PLWHA), the following specific principles should be applied to people who inject drugs:

- ART is as effective for people who inject drugs as for other people with HIV/AIDS.
- Given appropriate support, former and current users of injection drugs can adhere to and have equal success on ART.
- Current or past drug use should not be a criterion for deciding on who should receive ART.
- Special attention should be paid to the particular needs of former and current users of injection drugs, including those related to substance dependence, comorbidities and coinfections.
- A public health policy that acknowledges and addresses the need to treat both substance dependence and HIV/AIDS improves patient well-being, reduces stigma and promotes delivery of comprehensive, ethical medical care.
- The most effective response consists of a combination of prevention, care, treatment and support within a harm reduction framework.

- Provision of quality OST for opioid-dependent people who inject drugs is an important component of HIV/AIDS care and treatment, and is highly effective.
- A supportive environment, upholding the human rights and dignity of people who inject drugs and helping to expand and improve access to drug dependence treatment, should be ensured.
- Countries with HIV epidemics fuelled by IDU should respond immediately to the needs of people who inject drugs with preventive and treatment services.

Development of this treatment and care guide

This guide is designed to complement the global ART guidelines and is based on the WHO publications *Antiretroviral therapy for HIV infection in adults and adolescents* (2006) and the draft *HIV/AIDS treatment and care for injecting drug users, clinical protocol for the WHO European Region* (2006). A consultation and discussions were held with health-care workers, researchers and programme managers from the South-East Asia and Western Pacific Regions, and experiences were shared from scaling up ART and harm reduction services. The initial working group was convened in Kuala Lumpur, Malaysia and a first draft for regional adaptation was completed in August 2006. An online consultative process was then established to finalize the document. The final editing was done by WHO (WPRO and SEARO) and UNODC. This guide has been developed in recognition of the need for physicians, programme planners, other health-care workers, PLWHA and drug users to have one simplified, user-friendly reference guide for national adaptation on the management of HIV infection and ART for people who inject drugs.

Who is this guide for?

The guide is designed for primary care physicians who provide care and treatment to individuals infected with HIV through IDU. It may also be useful for other health-care providers such as nurses, pharmacists, addiction specialists and professionals in other health-related fields. Although some patients would have used injection drugs in the past and are not current users, many who require HIV treatment will continue to inject drugs. This guide is designed to provide a practical and detailed approach to ART and addiction treatment, although supplementary documents will be useful.

The content of this guide is aligned with other publications on HIV treatment and IDU released by the WHO HQ and the Regional Offices for the South-East Asia and Western Pacific Regions.

I. BACKGROUND AND GENERAL CONSIDERATIONS

1. Epidemiology of HIV and injecting drug use

Estimates suggest that by the end of 2003, there were approximately 13.2 million people worldwide who injected drugs, the majority (10.3 million [78%]) in developing and transitional countries. The number of people who inject drugs in South and South-East Asia was estimated at 3.3 million.[14] HIV epidemics in many parts of the world are driven by injection drug use (IDU) and sexual contact with those who inject drugs. It is estimated that at least 10% of all new infections in the world – a figure that rises to 30% when Africa is excluded – can be attributed to IDU and that approximately 3 million past and current people who inject drugs are living with HIV/AIDS.[15]

In most parts of the South-East Asia and Western Pacific Regions, HIV epidemics have been largely driven by IDU, although HIV transmission is also high among commercial sex workers and their clients. Indonesia, Malaysia, Myanmar, Thailand and Viet Nam are all estimated to have HIV prevalence rates of more than 20% among people who inject drugs; some regional estimates are as high as 70%.[14,16] In Indonesia, a country with one of the fastest-growing HIV epidemics in Asia, 51% of all newly reported HIV infections up to March 2006 occurred among people who inject drugs.[17] In China, it is estimated that over half of new HIV infections are occurring among the country's estimated 1.14 million registered drug users.[18] There are an estimated 288 000 drug users living with HIV/AIDS in China, accounting for 44% of all HIV cases.[19,20] Other countries in Asia, including Bangladesh, Lao PDR and the Philippines currently have low prevalence rates of HIV, although the risk environment is in place for a scenario of rapid HIV transmission among people who inject drugs. The countries most affected are primarily those where access to prevention, care and treatment are limited, needle and syringe programmes, and drug substitution therapy are not widely available (if not illegal), and law enforcement is the dominant response to drug use.

Explosive growth is one characteristic of IDU-driven HIV epidemics. In some cases, HIV prevalence among people who inject drugs has risen dramatically in just a few years.[21–23] IDU-driven HIV epidemics typically start with young, male and sexually active people who inject drugs. This is then followed by sexual transmission to male and female partners as well as to children through mother-to-child transmission (MTCT).

Sex work and IDU are closely linked in most settings. This sets up a particularly high-risk environment for HIV transmission and also has the potential to create an important "bridge" to the general population.[24] This has been well described in China, where female sex workers who became infected through IDU or through sexual contact with men who inject drugs subsequently transmitted

HIV to those in the general population.[25] A study from eastern India, which borders Nepal, Bangladesh and Bhutan, found that over 50% of men who inject drugs visited a commercial sex worker in the previous year and this has significant implications for cross-border transmission of HIV.[26] In Viet Nam, sex work and IDU have resulted in epidemic rates of sexually transmitted infections (STIs) and subsequent explosive outbreaks of HIV infection.[27] The increasing rates of HIV infection among non-injecting sex partners of people who inject drugs should also receive intensive prevention efforts. In Chennai, India, not only were HIV rates among female sex partners of people who inject drugs very high, but there was also an alarmingly low perception of HIV risk.[28] The transmission of HIV from males who inject drugs to the their female partners is compounded by an extreme imbalance of power in sexual relationships, which results in high vulnerability to HIV among females, as seen in Sichuan Province, China.[29]

The lack of access to prevention and treatment interventions (notably harm reduction), and high efficiency of bloodborne transmission of HIV through needle-sharing and sharing of other drug paraphernalia explain these explosive epidemics. An additional factor is the elevated level of viraemia characteristic of the first weeks and months after seroconversion, which may contribute to the high HIV transmission rates typical of these epidemics.[30]

2. Health and social consequences of injecting drug use

Substance dependence is a complex condition that has both physical and psychosocial components, and is associated with severe morbidity and a high risk of death. Substance dependence is a chronic, relapsing condition, which is difficult to control due to compulsive drug use and craving, leading to drug-seeking and repetitive use, even in the face of negative health and social consequences.[31] A number of medical, psychiatric and social problems are common among substance-dependent people around the world, which are important considerations in designing and delivering HIV/AIDS care.

2.1. Health problems

In addition to HIV, people who inject drugs have an increased incidence of other bloodborne infections and injecting-related health issues. If contaminated needles and syringes are shared, IDU can result in exposure to the viruses causing hepatitis B and C (HBV, HCV) as well as HIV. Other injecting-related health issues include the risk of overdose and a wide range of bacterial infections. Criminalization of IDU further exacerbates the severe social and health consequences, including high rates of incarceration, traumatic injury, STIs and tuberculosis (TB).

Some people who inject drugs have a long history of mental illness that has not been properly diagnosed or treated. There are some mental conditions that may result from, or be exacerbated by, the use of substances such as alcohol, cocaine and opioids.[32,33] These substances may also be used as a form of self-medication for symptoms of mental illness and substitute for effective treatment. A substantial increase in the frequency of major depression and suicide in HIV-positive people who inject drugs is apparent, even above the elevated rates associated with advanced HIV infection and AIDS.[34–36]

Common health problems among people who inject drugs include the following:

- infection with other bloodborne viruses, including HBV and HCV, which may lead to serious liver diseases including cirrhosis and hepatocellular carcinoma;
- injection-related bacterial infections, including septicaemia, bacterial endocarditis and osteomyelitis;
- local soft tissue and vascular injury, including skin abscesses and thrombophlebitis;
- TB, both pulmonary and extrapulmonary;
- psychiatric comorbidity including depression;
- overdose; and
- polysubstance dependence, including alcohol.

The above health problems are considered in more detail in Section III (Clinical management of HIV-infected people who inject drugs).

2.2. Social problems

Common perceptions that drug users do not adhere to antiretroviral therapy (ART) may overlook the confounding effects of social instability and marginalization, poverty, homelessness, unemployment, psychiatric morbidity, incarceration and poor patient–physician relationships. Harm reduction, general medical care, treatment for substance dependence, psychiatric treatment and psychosocial support should be integrated to optimize the care of HIV-infected people who inject drugs.

2.2.1. Stigma, discrimination and social marginalization

Drug use is a prevailing source of stigma and discrimination and, when coupled with being HIV-positive, people who inject drugs often face a double burden of stigma and social marginalization.[37] In some cases, the added stigma of sex work makes the situation even more difficult and may drive individuals to the margins of society.

- Stigma attached to drug use is often reinforced by the fact that using drugs is an illegal and covert activity, and that there is often no legal protection available to people who use drugs.
- Drug users often experience stigma and discrimination when they attend medical facilities and are therefore reluctant to attend.
- Fear of discrimination may discourage HIV-infected drug users from revealing their drug use to an HIV/AIDS care specialist, leading to a greater risk of misdiagnosis, or of pharmacological interactions between the HIV treatment regimens and substances used.
- Many people who inject drugs live on the economic and social fringes of society, and may be rejected by their families.
- People who are most vulnerable to the impact of poverty, racial discrimination, poor health, lack of education and employment are also those most vulnerable to drug use.
- Social problems and discrimination faced by people who are drug dependent and/or HIV-positive may in turn exacerbate drug use.

Stigma and discrimination should be considered and dealt with at the health sector level by the following means:

- Ensure that the human rights of people who inject drugs are respected, and that such people receive quality services that address their health needs, including ART.
- Ensure that health-care workers are aware of their own feelings and prejudices, and of the effect this may have on their patients, their professional performance and the successful outcome of drug dependence treatment and ART.
- Ensure that the facilities to engage people who inject drugs are welcoming and provide a friendly and supportive environment.
- Guarantee confidentiality of patients.
- Include specific reference to appropriate professional behaviour in relevant health service guidelines, protocols and staff regulations.
- Refer patients to other appropriate services to assist with social problems and the consequences of discriminatory practices, including education, housing, legal services, social work, etc.

2.2.2. Closed settings including prisons

The economic pressure of supporting drug dependence may result in criminal activity. This is in addition to the laws criminalizing drug possession, use and trafficking. Thus, a large proportion of drug users are periodically incarcerated. Many countries in Asia have some form of compulsory detoxification in the form of rehabilitation centres. These are abstinence-based facilities that do not employ evidence-based methods for drug dependence treatment. It is widely accepted that these approaches are ineffective as forms of drug treatment and can further produce a range of problems.

Problems associated with closed settings include:

- unsafe IDU with the risk of HBV, HCV and HIV transmission;
- an environment highly conducive to other communicable diseases, including TB, in particular, multidrug-resistant TB (MDR-TB);
- unprotected sex between prisoners, with the associated risk of HIV and other STI transmission;
- increased risk of overdose after release from prison;
- physical and sexual assault; and
- depression, anxiety and suicide.

Explosive HIV epidemics within prisons have been reported in a number of countries, and such epidemics can trigger or significantly impact on broader HIV epidemics.[38] Ensuring that HIV/AIDS prevention, care and treatment services are provided in prison, rehabilitation centres and other closed settings is a critical component for a public health response to HIV/AIDS. WHO has provided guidance on HIV prevention and treatment in prisons and other closed settings.[39,40] It is also extremely important to link individuals to services following release from closed settings to ensure continuity. Formal lines of communication between closed setting facilities, and health and addiction services should be established.

II. ORGANIZATION AND MANAGEMENT CONSIDERATIONS

1. Services for people who inject drugs

The organization of HIV prevention, care and treatment services, and their linkages to other services are important determinants of successful treatment for people who inject drugs. Four types of interrelated and linked services are crucial for the treatment of substance dependence and HIV/AIDS. These are:

- general medical care;
- harm reduction;
- drug dependence treatment; and
- psychosocial support.

The provision of ART through a programme of directly administered ART (DAART) may also improve outcomes in terms of viral suppression and treatment engagement.[41] Participants in a DAART programme would be expected to attend a clinic setting each day to consume at least one dose of their antiretroviral (ARV) drugs. This model of ART delivery is very resource intensive and may not be appropriate in all settings but does optimize adherence and clinical monitoring.

1.1. General medical care

WHO favours a multidisciplinary approach for the provision of care and treatment for PLWHA. The care team should have experience with drug dependence issues. A care team typically includes:

- clinician (physician or other medical practitioner);
- medical nurse;
- social worker;
- counselling staff; and
- substance dependence specialist(s) (e.g. addiction specialist and/or psychiatrist and/or psychologist).

The availability of substance dependence specialists, especially those experienced in illicit drugs, is limited in most countries. Psychiatrists and psychiatric services are not necessarily the most appropriate clinicians/institutions to provide substance dependence treatment. There is the risk of additional stigmatization of drug users because of their association with psychiatric services, particularly if they do not have psychiatric comorbidity. In many countries, general practitioners and other types of physicians manage drug dependence. WHO therefore recommends involving a multidisciplinary team that includes clinicians with training and experience in the management of drug dependence. The team should meet on a regular basis to review the status of people who inject drugs under its care, and work out case management plans with objectives and goals. A major challenge in delivering care to people who inject drugs is their need for multiple services concurrently to address both medical and psychosocial issues. Successful programmes must be accessible to the population, free of charge, provided in a non-judgemental manner and tailored to the individual's needs.

The person receiving care must necessarily be an integral part of setting the programme's objectives and goals.

Medical care should be comprehensive in order to address HIV infection. In addition, people who inject drugs require:

- treatment adherence support;
- drug (opioid) substitution therapy (OST);
- other substance dependence treatment;
- reduction of risk behaviours, including both drug use and sexual behaviours;
- support for sexual partners;
- support for social matters (through social services); and
- health education.

HIV treatment programmes should be linked with harm reduction services to facilitate enrolment and retention of people who inject drugs, and to ensure that those on treatment can readily access risk reduction advice and counselling. Harm reduction strategies, including drug substitution therapy, can limit the medical and psychosocial complications of drug use, and facilitate HIV care by stabilizing behaviours. Continuity of care can be strengthened by good referral systems between different health services; between health services and community organizations, IDU networks and families; and between institutional, home-based and community care. Outreach strategies are a vital component, forming strong links with community-based organizations representing affected groups, and utilizing peer educators and counsellors drawn from these groups.

Treatment programmes for HIV-positive people who inject drugs need to incorporate general medical care for clinical conditions that commonly affect such people. The ready availability of such services will enhance a programme's credibility, while their absence will signal a lack of concern for the immediate needs of people who inject drugs.[42]

1.2. Harm reduction

Harm reduction interventions reduce the adverse health, social and economic consequences of psychoactive substance use for individual drug users, their families and their communities. Comprehensive harm reduction programmes can reduce new HIV infections among people who inject drugs.[43–45]

WHO has a long tradition of working in HIV/AIDS prevention, care and treatment for people who inject drugs and prisoners. This work is guided by a broad range of WHO and United Nations resolutions, commitments, policies, position papers and technical documents, and is now solidly evidenced-based on the concept of harm reduction. The *1974 Report of the WHO Expert Committee on Drug Dependence* statement, which pre-dates the HIV/AIDS epidemic, nonetheless provides the rationale for WHO's public health approach to addressing drug-related problems within a harm reduction framework, advocating that programmes should be primarily concerned with preventing and reducing problems related to drug use rather than preventing drug use itself.

In May 2003, the 56th World Health Assembly endorsed the *WHO Global Health Sector Strategy (GHSS) for HIV/AIDS 2003–2007*. The Strategy lists the core components of a comprehensive health sector response to HIV/AIDS, including *"promoting harm reduction among injecting drug users, such as wide access to sterile injecting equipment, and drug dependence treatment and outreach services to help reduce frequency of injecting drug use"*. The key components of an effective harm reduction package targeting drug users include:

- community outreach, with a focus on peer approaches;
- behaviour change communication, including risk reduction information;
- access to clean needles and syringes as well as their safe disposal;
- drug dependence treatment, particularly OST;
- HIV testing and counselling (voluntary and confidential, and provider initiated);
- prevention of sexual transmission through interventions such as providing condoms, and STI prevention and treatment;
- HIV/AIDS care and treatment, including ART;
- primary health care, including hepatitis B vaccination, vein and abscess/ulcer care, overdose management; and
- supportive policy and legislative environment.

WHO has recently renewed its commitment to providing universal access to HIV/AIDS prevention, care and treatment for all who need it. As part of that commitment, harm reduction is a priority intervention. WHO's harm reduction work is guided by a number of technical papers and policy briefs.

TECHNICAL PAPERS

- *Effectiveness of sterile needle and syringe programming in reducing HIV/AIDS among injecting drug users*[46]
  http://www.who.int/hiv/pub/prev_care/en/effectivenesssterileneedle.pdf

- *Effectiveness of community-based outreach in preventing HIV/AIDS among injecting drug users*[47]
  http://www.who.int/hiv/pub/prev_care/en/evidenceforactionreprint2004.pdf

- *Effectiveness of drug dependence treatment in preventing HIV among injecting drug users*[48]
  http://www.who.int/hiv/pub/idu/en/drugdependencefinaldraft.pdf

POLICY BRIEFS

- *Provision of sterile injecting equipment to reduce HIV transmission*[49]
  http://www.who.int/hiv/pub/advocacy/en/provisionofsterileen.pdf

- *Reduction of HIV transmission through drug-dependence treatment*[50]
  http://www.who.int/hiv/pub/advocacy/en/drugdependencetreatmenten.pdf

- *Reduction of HIV transmission in prisons*[51]
  http://www.who.int/hiv/pub/advocacy/en/transmissionprisonen.pdf

- *Reduction of HIV transmission through outreach*[52]
  http://www.who.int/hiv/pub/advocacy/en/throughoutreachen.pdf

- *Antiretroviral therapy and injecting drug users*[53]
  http://www.who.int/hiv/pub/prev_care/arvidu.pdf

1.2.1. Harm reduction programmes

The adoption of harm reduction programmes varies considerably throughout South and South-East Asia as does their organization and modes of service delivery. In China, there has been a concerted effort to increase needle and syringe availability in some communities.[54] A common feature is the training of staff (e.g. social workers, counsellors and outreach workers) who have access to drug-using populations, and are able to work in a non-judgemental manner and in an environment of trust. In Indonesia, the scale up of harm reduction strategies took a major turn in 2006. As of mid-2006, there were 91 needle and syringe programmes in the country, seven methadone clinics (including one inside a prison in Bali) and increasing access to care, support and treatment, including ART, for people who inject drugs.[55]

In addition to the critical and proven HIV prevention strategies of needle and syringe programmes and condom distribution, harm reduction services should be involved in:

- HIV/AIDS treatment delivery where feasible;
- ART adherence support, including maintaining follow up with people who inject drugs and who drop out of care;
- providing low-threshold (easy to enter or accessible) entry points for both HIV/AIDS and drug dependence treatment;
- providing information on safer drug use and HIV prevention, potential interactions between the non-medical use of psychoactive drugs and HIV/AIDS treatment and ART, including how to manage ART-related side-effects;
- referrals to other harm reduction services, including drug dependence treatment programmes, community support services and other health-care services;
- conducting outreach to people who inject drugs for HIV testing, counselling, care and treatment; and
- providing direct ART services, including prescribing and clinical monitoring, where appropriate.

1.3. Drug dependence treatment and opioid substitution therapy

HIV and drug dependence are not isolated problems, but influence the progression of each other. There are a variety of treatment modalities for drug dependence, including drug-free residential therapy, outpatient counselling-based treatment, and medication-assisted substitution and detoxification for opioid dependence.[56,57] Effective treatment options using evidence-based counselling approaches for dependence on cocaine and amphetamine-type stimulants (ATS) should also be offered. Medication-assisted therapy for cocaine and ATS dependence may be of benefit, although substitution therapy for non-opioid dependence is much less developed and generally unavailable outside of research protocols.[58] Given the chronic and relapsing nature of substance dependence, detoxification alone is seldom effective in producing long-term and sustained change.[59]

Treatment of drug dependence, in particular through OST, provides many benefits in the prevention and treatment of HIV/AIDS by:

- improving access to HIV care and treatment and general health care;
- retaining active drug users in treatment;
- reducing the transmission of HIV, viral hepatitis and bacterial infections;

- decreasing the need for hospitalization;
- improving and facilitating adherence and follow up of patients on ART;
- reducing illicit opioid use;
- reducing criminal activity;
- decreasing deaths due to overdose;
- cutting down on behaviours with a high risk of HIV transmission; and
- improving social integration.

The benefits of substitution therapy programmes can be maximized by:

- prescribing methadone or buprenorphine in doses that effectively prevent craving and reduce drug use;
- orientating programmes towards maintenance rather than abstinence;
- offering counselling, assessment and treatment for psychiatric comorbidity and social problems;
- using evidence-based strategies such as motivational interviewing or contingency management to assist patients in reducing the use of additional drugs; and
- ensuring ready access to services, including convenient geographical location and opening hours, and affordable cost.

Where substitution therapy is available, consideration should be given to offering HIV/AIDS medical care and dispensing ART at the same site from which drug substitution therapy is dispensed.[60] This approach can:

- achieve maximal levels of treatment supervision and improve adherence;
- reduce the risk of developing ARV drug resistance;
- facilitate the management of interactions between methadone and HIV/AIDS medications; and
- provide the opportunity to administer DAART to patients attending daily to receive methadone (a second "take-home" ARV dose is usually needed).

1.4. Psychosocial support

Concurrent services that address both the biomedical needs and the psychosocial issues of people who inject drugs are essential.[61] A wide range of psychosocial support services should be available and accessed according to the needs of the patient, including:

- support services for adherence to ART;
- psychological support/counselling, group therapy for people who inject drugs and family members;
- peer support groups;
- educational programmes;
- psychiatric/psychological services for assessment and management of mental health disorders; and
- social/welfare services to deal with problems related to housing, employment, finances, legal issues, discrimination and other issues.

People who injected drugs in the past often have unique success in educating and motivating people who currently inject drugs, including:

- accessing the hard-to-reach sectors of the population and referring them to effective prevention, care and treatment services;
- preparing people who inject drugs for treatment, such as advising them on the potential side-effects associated with ART; and
- supporting people who inject drugs to adhere to ART and other treatment.

The inclusion of former injecting drug users in education and outreach programmes requires adequate training and supervision, as well as close monitoring, as there is a high risk of relapse to illicit drug use for these peer workers.

2. Models of comprehensive HIV/AIDS care for people who inject drugs

HIV/AIDS care and treatment, including ART, should be delivered as part of a comprehensive care model. Combining or integrating HIV/AIDS and substance dependence services provides opportunities for HIV prevention, enhances adherence to both HIV/AIDS and substance dependence treatment, and provides better overall care for HIV-infected people who inject drugs. A comprehensive service develops expertise in effectively treating substance dependence and providing HIV care. There are a range of models for effectively combining HIV prevention, care and treatment with substance dependence treatment. One model would be to provide on-site HIV/AIDS medical care for people who inject drugs in a substance dependence treatment facility. Alternatively, a substance dependence treatment component could be integrated with HIV/AIDS services.

A variant of the on-site model is mobile health care that may be linked to an HIV/AIDS medical care centre, a substance dependence treatment facility or a harm reduction service. Mobile services can provide HIV and STI screening, HIV/AIDS treatment, and referrals to substance dependence treatment, mental health and other services. Primary care services can also be offered for both drug dependence management and HIV/AIDS care through general practitioners or office-based practices.

The potential effectiveness of the models will depend largely on the overall infrastructure and organization of the health-care system. Where specialized departments (for example, drug treatment centres and departments of internal medicine) exist, linkages between these departments and the case to be managed should be common practice.

3. Care within closed settings

Reaching people who inject drugs in prisons and other closed settings is crucial because these facilities exacerbate the risks of HIV infection and drug dependence.[62] People in closed settings should receive the same package of services as those who are not in these settings, including ART. Treatment for HIV/AIDS and/or substance dependence may have begun prior to entry into a closed setting and this must be continued. Programmes have shown that ART can be successfully administered in prisons.[63,64]

Providing prevention, treatment and harm reduction interventions in prison to people who inject drugs benefits individual inmates as well as the community at large.[65,66] In Asia, there is currently only one comprehensive harm reduction service inside a prison and this is located in Bali, Indonesia. This programme provides bleach and condoms, care and treatment (including ART) and methadone to prisoners.[67] The Indonesian National AIDS Commission has recently decided to extend such services to the other 95 prisons in the country. Despite this advancement, most countries have been slow to recognize the serious risks of HIV epidemics within closed settings. A comprehensive programme in a closed setting should include:

- information, education and communication on HIV/AIDS;
- voluntary counselling and testing;
- distribution of condoms;
- access to sterile needles and syringes (and where this is not feasible, bleach or other disinfectants);
- OST;
- clinical management in prisons of drug-dependent prisoners at a standard equivalent to that in the local community;
- care and treatment services related to HIV/AIDS (including ART), hepatitis and TB; and
- follow-through care with links to community services.

Continuity of care for HIV-infected drug users released from prison needs to be ensured. There is a need for strong links to be established among closed settings, drug dependence "treatment" centres, prisons, labour camps and other centres of detention, as many drug-dependent people will move back and forth between the community and such settings.

It is crucial that programmes in closed settings:

- ensure continuity of services between the community and detention;
- be approached as opportunities for HIV prevention, care and treatment; and
- be monitored and evaluated using a range of indicators covering drug use, HIV and social issues.

WHO and UNODC have provided guidance on HIV prevention and treatment in prisons and other closed settings.[39,40]

III. CLINICAL MANAGEMENT OF HIV-INFECTED PEOPLE WHO INJECT DRUGS

1. Initial patient evaluation

Care for HIV-positive people who inject drugs must address substance use and dependence, psychological and social issues, and medical complications associated with IDU. As noted above, WHO favours a multidisciplinary approach for the provision of HIV care and treatment. The care team should have experience with drug dependence issues, although such expertise may not be readily available in many countries. Establishing programmes that offer ART to people who inject drugs should not be delayed because of a lack of expertise, and the absence of such experts should not be used as a barrier to starting ART in those who inject drugs. The ultimate goal should be to form a care team that includes providers who have acquired substance dependence expertise.

1.1. Screening and assessment for substance dependence

Standardized screening and assessment tools should be used for the purpose of screening for, and initial evaluation of, substance use and substance dependence. Several validated and standardized dependence screening and assessment instruments are available. Preferred screening and assessment instruments are suggested below. The use of any screening and assessment tool must be preceded by voluntary and fully informed consent, and an explanation of why it is necessary for the service/clinician to have an understanding of the individual's substance use and associated problems.

1.1.1 Screening

Those who admit to the use of substances (or those who do not but have clinical signs of drug use) should be interviewed further. Initial screening should consist of a combination of screening observations, interviews and use of standardized instruments. The goal of such screening is to establish substance use patterns and suitability for substance dependence treatment.

Patients who use drugs may or may not be substance dependent. This has significant implications for future management, hence it is crucial to assess drug dependence. Non-specialized staff can administer a rapid and simple initial assessment of drug dependence. It is based on a ten-question questionnaire, adapted from the *International Classification of Disease, 10th revision (ICD-10) symptom checklist for mental disorders.*

1.1.2 Assessment

Typically, a substance use and substance dependence assessment includes a complete history, including that of substance use, previous treatment for substance use and a physical examination. During the initial meetings it may be difficult to ask specific questions around illicit drug use, given that the use of these substances is illegal and there is a real risk of detention in most Asian countries. It is extremely important to gain the trust of the potential client and ensure confidentiality. As a first step, the assessment should include the following:

- Describe the drug dependence treatment services that are available (detoxification programme, OST, 12-step programme, etc.).
- Ask the client if they would be interested in accessing any of these services.
- Explain that access to the addiction service will necessitate an evaluation of drug dependence and explain what the assessment would involve.
- If the client chooses to be assessed, proceed with the substance dependence assessment.

A substance use and treatment history will include:

- substances used (including alcohol);
- modes of drug administration (including injecting use);
- age at first use as well as recent and current use;
- changes in drug effects over time;
- daily dosing including dose at one time and the number of times per day;
- history of overdose and withdrawal;
- periods of abstinence and attempts to quit;
- complications of substance use (e.g. skin infections); and
- treatment history, including previous treatments for drug dependence, types and outcomes of treatments.

A physical examination may indicate substance dependence and/or complications associated with substance use. The physical complications of opioid or other drug dependence should be identified and addressed as part of the overall treatment plan.

A standardized assessment tool can be used to assess the severity of the addiction and suitability for the range of drug treatment options. A potential tool is the *Addiction Severity Index (ASI), European version 6 (EuropASI6)*.

In addition, risk-taking behaviour with regard to bloodborne diseases can be documented using a standardized instrument such as the *Bloodborne virus transmission risk assessment questionnaire (BBV-TRAQ),* Turning Point Alcohol and Drug Centre Inc., 1988, though the questionnaire is rather more a research tool, time-consuming and will not be acceptable in many clinical settings.

1.2. Initial evaluation of a patient's HIV/AIDS status

Initial evaluation of the HIV/AIDS status of people who inject drugs is no different from that of non-injectors. Offering HIV counselling and testing and information should be a routine procedure in health-care settings dealing with patients who inject drugs. Health-care providers should explain to patients the reasons for offering the test and the importance of knowing the results to allow for appropriate clinical management. However, everyone has the right to refuse the test. Initial assessment of the HIV status should include the following:

- HIV pre-test counselling, education and information;
- serological test (typically rapid HIV tests and/or enzyme-linked immunosorbent assay [ELISA]) for HIV antibodies following the national testing algorithms; and
- post-test counselling, including information on reducing risky behaviour, irrespective of whether the HIV test is positive or negative.

Clinical evaluation of an HIV-infected person is necessary to develop a strategy for management. Evaluation includes:

- presenting symptoms;
- physical examination including height and weight;
- mental health and social assessment;
- preparedness for treatment (what are the patient's beliefs about ART, how will taking medications fit in with their routine);
- routine laboratory assessment – complete blood count (haemoglobin [Hb], white blood cell [WBC] count, differential WBC count, platelets); with full renal function tests, serum electrolytes, liver function tests (alanine aminotransferase [ALT]), if available at the ART clinic level;
- history of contraception use and a pregnancy test for women, particularly if efavirenz (EFV) and tenofovir disoproxil fumarate (TDF) are considered;
- assessment for HBV and HCV infection;
- screening for TB; and
- testing for other STIs.

The absence of the following desirable and optimal tests cannot be a barrier to starting ART:

- CD4 lymphocyte count to determine the severity of immunodeficiency (if available)
- Viral load testing (if available) to monitor the response to ART.

Since many people who inject drugs present for care at an advanced stage of HIV infection, it is important to thoroughly evaluate new patients for active opportunistic infections (OIs). The initial history and physical examination will usually identify common infections. These conditions should not be interpreted as exclusion criteria for ART, but viewed individually as situations in which clinical judgement should be used. Initial evaluation should be followed by treatment of OIs and other conditions as indicated. Furthermore, the use of isoniazid and co-trimoxazole prophylaxis should be considered as in individuals who do not inject drugs.

1.3. Psychosocial assessment

Mental health comorbidities are also common among people who inject drugs. It is estimated that between 25% and 50% of drug users also have a comorbid mental health problem.[68–70] The provision of appropriate mental health support, comprising both psychiatric (e.g. for mood disorders, psychotic illnesses) and psychological inputs (e.g. anxiety management, behavioural therapy), is an important component of drug treatment services.

Adherence to ART may be enhanced by providing antidepressant treatment if the patient is found to be clinically depressed.[71] Good liaison models should be developed to enhance the care of individuals with mental health disorders. Clinicians working in mental health should be aware of the potential drug interactions between psychotropic medications and ARVs, particularly with EFV.

Social factors may have a profound effect on the uptake and sustainability of ART among people who inject drugs, and overwhelm some of the best care and treatment programmes. In resource-limited settings this is a particular challenge, as profound poverty, homelessness and a lack of financial security are commonplace. Add to this a lack of family and community support, and serious life events including incarceration and violence, the prospects for successful HIV care and treatment are greatly reduced. Social support is therefore critical to the ultimate success of ART.

2. Managing opioid dependence

Despite polysubstance use in many regions, the management of opioid dependence remains the major focus of OST and other harm reduction strategies. The absence of OST, however, cannot be a barrier to access for people who inject drugs to ART, nor to the provision of other drug treatment approaches. The following considerations are key to the effective management of opioid dependence:

- Successful drug dependence management will improve outcomes in terms of improved CD4 counts and adherence to ART.
- Although OST is not universally available, the lack of access to OST should not preclude active drug users from accessing ART.
- Stabilization of opioid-dependent people who inject drugs through OST is a key component of successful HIV/AIDS treatment.
- A principle of OST is to provide a supportive therapeutic environment in order to stabilize the lifestyle of the individual.
- Staff in substance dependence services need regular ongoing contact with people who inject drugs, whether or not the individual is being treated with OST.
- Treatment for opioid dependence should be accessible (geographically and at suitable times), free of charge, user-friendly, confidential and free of legal harassment.
- Treatment for opioid dependence should include a range of evidence-informed treatment options and be viewed as a vital public health intervention.

Given the range of treatment interventions and the skills mix available within a multidisciplinary team, staff working in drug dependence treatment services need to have extensive and ongoing contact with people who inject drugs, even if OST is not an option. Therefore, there is a need to train and educate drug dependence staff in the issues related to HIV management. Each service should also explore options around dispensing ART in novel settings such as needle exchange or drop-in/outreach centres (centres where people can come to without an appointment for information about health, drugs, social services, etc.). Confidentiality and assurance that patients will not be legally harassed are essential while offering treatment.

2.1. Opioid substitution therapies

Effective pharmacotherapy is available for opioid dependence. Pharmacotherapeutic options include maintenance therapy with the opioid agonist **methadone** given orally; maintenance therapy with the partial opioid agonist **buprenorphine** given sublingually, or a combination of sublingual **buprenorphine** and **naloxone**; and the use of methadone/buprenorphine (or **clonidine**) to treat withdrawal/drug detoxification to facilitate entry into drug-free or antagonist treatment approaches.[72]

The two main medications used for OST – methadone and buprenorphine – have been included in the WHO list of essential medicines since 2005, although their availability may be limited in parts of Asia. OST dispensed on a daily basis can promote frequent contact with staff and may improve access and adherence to ART.

2.1.1. Methadone

Methadone is a synthetic opioid and is the most common medication used for substitution therapy of opioid dependence. The global number of persons with opioid dependence receiving prescribed methadone is estimated to be over half a million and is increasing in almost all regions of the world. Originally implemented in the United States, Australia and Western Europe, methadone maintenance treatment is expanding eastwards to Central and Eastern Europe, to the Eastern Mediterranean Region and to Asia. Methadone is also being used for the treatment of opioid dependence in Argentina, Canada, China, Indonesia, Iran, New Zealand, Thailand and other countries. One of the most aggressive scale-ups of methadone clinics is currently under way in China where the first eight clinics were opened in 2004, and an additional 128 clinics had been approved in 2005.[73] It is estimated that up to one million people will be receiving methadone maintenance treatment in China by 2010.

Doses of methadone in different programmes range from 20 to 150 mg per day and sometimes higher. Doses of 60–120 mg are more effective in achieving retention in treatment and reducing illicit drug use than lower dosages. Clinical trials have demonstrated the effectiveness of methadone maintenance therapy for the treatment of opioid dependence and prevention of HIV. Such evidence is summarized in WHO documents.[48,74]

2.1.2. Buprenorphine

More recently, buprenorphine has been used for both detoxification and maintenance of opioid-dependent individuals.

The global number of persons with opioid dependence receiving prescribed buprenorphine is estimated to be 200 000 and increasing in practically all regions. In 2005, buprenorphine maintenance treatment was available in 29 countries. The greatest level of experience with buprenorphine has been in France where buprenorphine treatment for heroin dependence has been widely available through general practitioners since 1995. By 2001, approximately 74 000 patients per year were on buprenorphine treatment in France, while 9600 were treated with methadone.[75]

The effective maintenance dose of buprenorphine ranges between 12 and 34 mg with an average daily dose of 16 mg. Due to its partial antagonist properties, buprenorphine is less likely than methadone to cause overdose. In addition, it appears to offer a slightly smoother withdrawal during detoxification. Buprenorphine has a higher affinity for the opioid receptors than nearly all other opioid agonist drugs. In addition, its partial rather than full agonist properties can lead to a precipitated withdrawal if administered after an opioid-dependent patient has been given an opioid agonist medication. Therefore, caution should be exercised in giving buprenophrine to patients taking morphine derivatives for pain. Buprenorphine is a sublingual preparation and care must be taken while dispensing as the tablets may be crushed and injected,[76] leading to the potential sharing of injecting equipment.[77] A number of clinical trials have demonstrated the effectiveness of buprenorphine maintenance therapy for the treatment of opioid dependence and this evidence is summarized in WHO documents.[50,78]

2.2. Retention in treatment

One of the best predictors of outcome in the management of drug dependence is retention in treatment. OST programmes are more successful in retaining participants in treatment than are detoxification and drug-free programmes. OST is therefore an ideal modality for the delivery of ART to HIV-positive people who inject drugs (evidently, if the drug in question is an opioid). All drug services should strive towards establishing methadone or buprenorphine maintenance therapy in order to improve treatment outcomes in their HIV-positive clients who inject opioid drugs. People who inject opioid drugs are less likely to receive ART if they are not enrolled in such a programme.[79]

In conjunction with methadone maintenance therapy, DAART should be considered because:

- it results in a significant number of patients achieving maximum viral suppression;
- it achieves higher levels of viral suppression than those injecting drug users receiving either standard care or treatment adherence support; and
- it minimizes the possible negative impact of ART on the daily routine of those who inject drugs.

2.3. Multidisciplinary approach

The management of drug-dependent individuals involves a multidisciplinary approach aimed at reducing harm resulting from the use of illicit drugs. While OST has been proven to be the most effective approach, it may not be available in all jurisdictions, some drug users do not inject opioids and some individuals may continue to use illicit drugs while receiving OST. Drug services should respond to the needs of people who inject drugs in line with the local and national policies and procedures. Government agencies, nongovernmental organizations (NGOs) and community groups should assist in the delivery of services. A range of interventions for people who inject drugs has evolved; from total abstinence to the provision of safe heroin for injection.[80]

In addition to the provision of OST, the range of treatment and management options includes the following:

- For patients not receiving OST, detoxification with or without antagonist medication (e.g. naltrexone)
- Self-help groups or peer support programmes
- Therapeutic communities including residential drug-free rehabilitation programmes of varying lengths (from 3 to 15 months), and group or individual psychotherapy and vocational training
- Residential rehabilitation including short-term residential programmes for 6–8 weeks
- Vocational training.

Psychological interventions are also important options for drug dependence and can be offered with or without OST. Psychotherapeutic modalities include the following:

- Cognitive–behavioural therapy (CBT): time-limited, structured, goal-oriented psychological intervention focusing on the problems of the drug user entering treatment. The therapy identifies the determinants or high-risk situations leading to drug use and allows the drug user to relearn appropriate coping skills, leading to a healthier lifestyle. CBT may be offered in short-term or extended programmes.[81]
- Motivational interviewing: stimulating and enhancing an individual's resolution to change.
- Contingency management: an intervention that reinforces or rewards appropriate positive behaviour. The reward may be in the form of vouchers that have a monetary value.[82, 83]
- Combination models: designed to integrate several interventions into a comprehensive approach. The elements include individual counselling, CBT, motivational interviewing, family education groups, urine testing and participation in a 12-step programme.[84]
- Relapse prevention: these strategies are aimed at maintaining abstinence and include medical or psychological interventions.

2.4. Detoxification programmes

Detoxification (medically supervised withdrawal) from opioids is an initial component of some treatment programmes but should never be considered as a treatment for opioid dependence on its own. Because opioid dependence is a chronic, relapsing condition, detoxification alone will not be effective in the long term as the majority of patients will relapse to drug use following detoxification if there are no subsequent interventions.

Detoxification should be individualized in order to provide supervised withdrawal from drug(s) of dependence, and reduce to a minimum the severity of withdrawal symptoms and seriousness of medical complications. Other considerations include the following:

- Reduction in methadone and buprenorphine doses should be negotiated with the drug user, depending on the emergence of withdrawal symptoms.

- Access to psychological support should be available throughout the detoxification period.
- Detoxification for opioid-dependent individuals can be carried out by tapering the doses of different medications.

MEDICATION	INITIAL DOSE	MAXIMUM DOSE	REDUCTION RATE	DURATION OF DETOXIFICATION
Buprenorphine	4–6 mg daily	12 mg per day	2 mg per day	5–8 days
Methadone	20–30 mg daily	40 mg per day	5 mg on alternate days	2–3 weeks
Clonidine	75–300 mcg daily in divided doses	900 mcg per day in divided doses	150 mcg per day	5–8 days

- When used appropriately, these medications can produce safe and less uncomfortable withdrawal; however, the majority of participants will relapse to opioid use after withdrawal, regardless of the method used.
- Detoxification programmes can provide entry points for ART delivery.

NOTE:

- To be effective, the patient must receive an appropriate dose of buprenorphine. Because of its antagonist effects, too high an initial dose of buprenorphine can induce opioid withdrawal. However, too low a dose will not relieve withdrawal symptoms.
- To provide adequate control of withdrawal symptoms but avoid the risk of overdose, especially in the first days of treatment, methadone can be given in divided doses. Withdrawal symptoms will commence as the dose is reduced; the more rapid the reduction, the greater the severity of the withdrawal symptoms.
- Clonidine can cause drowsiness, dizziness and profound postural hypotension even at low doses. It is important to take the patient's blood pressure before administering clonidine and throughout treatment, and modify the dosage if sustained hypotension occurs.

3. Managing non-opioid dependence (including cocaine and ATS)

While it is estimated that there are now over 13 million people who inject drugs worldwide, not all inject opioids. Other drugs, such as alcohol, sedatives, cocaine and ATS can also produce dependence. In addition, these substances can increase the risk of HIV transmission via unsafe injection practices or by increasing other behaviours such as unsafe sexual practices.[85–87] At present, there is no proven, effective substitution therapy for non-opioid drug dependence, although dexamphetamine has been prescribed to amphetamine users in the United Kingdom and Australia.[88] A number of promising pharmacotherapies for the treatment of cocaine dependence are under investigation as is cocaine vaccine. However, it is critical that services attempt to respond to the needs of non-opioid users.

Challenges faced in the provision of ART to cocaine and ATS users are similar to those faced by programmes dealing with active opioid users or those operating in situations where OST is not available. With the exception of substitution treatments for opioid dependence, the range of treatment options for non-opioid dependence is similar to those given above. There are, however, some further considerations in relation to medical management and psychological interventions, as follows:

- Acute medical detoxification from cocaine and ATS focuses on psychiatric symptom relief associated with prolonged sleep deprivation and withdrawal symptoms.
- Acute withdrawal problems are typically dealt with in the first 3–5 days post-cessation. However, particularly in individuals with comorbid medical or psychiatric problems, these can last up to two weeks.
- Detoxification should only form one part of a broader drug dependence treatment response.
- ATS use in general (and methamphetamine use in particular) has been associated with poor treatment engagement and high rates of drop-out and relapse.

3.1. Symptoms experienced and medications used

- Agitation and acute depression often follow cessation of cocaine or ATS use, and may require the use of a minor tranquillizer such as diazepam for a short period.
- Psychotic symptoms such as paranoia and sleep deprivation often develop with prolonged stimulant use, and may require antipsychotic medication.
- Palpitations and restlessness may benefit from the use of a beta-blocker such as **propranolol,** which has been shown to improve treatment retention and decrease cocaine use among those with severe withdrawal symptoms.[89] It should not be used in the presence of ongoing cocaine use.

3.2. Other interventions

Although there is no proven substitution therapy available for stimulant injectors, drug dependence services have regular and ongoing contact with these groups of patients. The psychological interventions mentioned above also have proven benefits in the treatment of cocaine and ATS use/dependence. CBT, a community reinforcement approach, contingency management and 12-step programmes have all been used for the treatment of cocaine and ATS dependence. [90-92]

4. Monitoring and evaluating effectiveness

Monitoring the effectiveness of the substance dependence treatment can be achieved through a number of means:

- Care planning is particularly informative; regular review by the case manager or physician is instrumental in achieving better outcomes.
- Care plans can set out short-, medium- and long-term goals for the individual. Monitoring how well these goals are met gives an indication of progress.
- Patient records are an essential element for documenting good practices and informing evaluation. They cover information on:
    - assessment results;
    - treatment plan;
    - daily dosages;
    - side-effects of prescribed medicines;
    - regimens used (including take-home doses);
    - medical care;
    - psychological and psychiatric care;
    - social care;
    - laboratory findings;
    - clinical observations;
    - programme compliance observations;
    - circumstances of leaving/terminating treatment;
    - agreement for terminating treatment; and
    - arrangements for after-care.
- The use of standardized instruments such as the Addiction Severity Index (ASI) allows progress to be monitored on a more formal basis.
- Screening of individuals for illicit drug use using urine analysis (if available) can give an indication of the response to the substance dependence treatment. In such cases, strict confidentiality is critical as in some regions this information may be used by law enforcement agencies to convict those in treatment programmes.
- Drug screening is not a necessary prerequisite and should only be undertaken with informed consent; a positive urine specimen should not be used as a criterion for terminating treatment.

5. Managing ART in HIV-infected people who inject drugs

Initiation of ART is never an emergency. Patients should be well informed, motivated and have had potential barriers to adherence addressed. Health-care providers should give information (preferably written, in the appropriate language and consistent with the literacy level) about ART to all patients and their families prior to initiation of treatment. Initiation of ART in HIV-infected people who inject drugs should follow the current recommendations (Table 1).

For complete details on treatment recommendations, refer to the WHO document *Antiretroviral therapy for HIV infection in adults and adolescents in resource-limited settings: towards universal access. Recommendations for a public health approach*, 2006 revision.[93]

TABLE 1: RECOMMENDATIONS FOR INITIATING ART IN HIV-INFECTED PATIENTS

WHO CLINICAL STAGING	CD4 TESTING NOT AVAILABLE	CD4 TESTING AVAILABLE
1	Do not treat	Treat if CD4 count is below 200 cells/mm^3 [a]
2	Do not treat[b]	
3	Treat	Consider treatment if CD4 count is below 350 cells/mm^3 [a,c,d] and initiate ART before CD4 count drops below 200 cells/mm^3 [e]
4	Treat	Treat irrespective of CD4 cell count [a]

Source: *Antiretroviral therapy for HIV infection in adults and adolescents in resource-limited settings: towards universal access. Recommendations for a public health approach.* Geneva, WHO, 2006:17.

a CD4 cell count advisable to assist with determining the need for immediate therapy in situations such as pulmonary TB and severe bacterial infections, which may occur at any CD4 level.
b A total lymphocyte count (TLC) of 1200 cells/mm³ or less can be substituted for the CD4 count when the latter is unavailable and mild HIV disease exists. It is not useful in asymptomatic patients. Thus, in the absence of CD4 cell counts and TLC, patients with WHO adult clinical stage 2 should not be treated.
c Initiation of ART is recommended in all HIV-infected pregnant women with WHO clinical stage 3 disease and CD4 counts below 350 cells/mm³.
d Initiation of ART is recommended for all HIV-infected patients with CD4 counts below 350 cells/mm³ and pulmonary TB or severe bacterial infection.
e The precise level of CD4 cell count above 200 cells/mm³ at which ART should be started has not been established.

While the CD4 count is the most important indicator for initiation of therapy, monitoring of treatment effects with plasma viral load is useful. However, attaining a baseline viral load is not necessary before starting therapy.

The decision to initiate ART in adults and adolescents is based on clinical and immunological assessment. In many resource-limited settings, only clinical staging will be available to guide the decision on when to start ART. The process of initiating ART involves assessment of patient readiness to commence therapy and an understanding of its implications (lifelong therapy, adherence, toxicities). Access to nutritional and psychosocial support, and family and peer support groups is important when making decisions about initiation of ART.

CD4 testing not available

In the absence of CD4 testing, all patients with WHO stage 3 and 4 disease should start ART, while those with WHO stage 1 and 2 disease should be monitored carefully, with a clinical review at a minimum of three-monthly intervals and at any time new symptoms develop. Availability of CD4 counts is not a prerequisite for starting ART and absence of or poor access to CD4 testing cannot be a barrier to the initiation of ART. Consider starting treatment for persons with WHO stage 2 disease and TLC <1200 cells/mm^3.

For complete details on monitoring, refer to the *WHO consultation on technical and operational recommendations for scale-up of laboratory services and monitoring HIV antiretroviral therapy in resource-limited settings*, September 2005.[94]

CD4 testing available

The optimum time to commence ART is before patients become unwell or present with their first OI. Immunological monitoring (CD4 testing) is the ideal way to approach this situation. A baseline CD4 cell count not only guides the decision on when to initiate ART but is also essential if CD4 counts will be used to monitor ART.[95-100]

The benchmark threshold that marks a substantially increased risk of clinical disease progression is a CD4 cell count of 200 cells/mm^3. Although it is never too late to initiate ART, patients should preferably begin therapy before the CD4 cell count drops to 200 cells/mm^3 or below. The optimum time to initiate ART in those with a CD4 cell count of 200–350 cells/mm^3 is unknown. Patients with CD4 cell counts in this range require regular clinical and immunological evaluation.

Initiation of ART is recommended for all patients with pulmonary TB or severe bacterial infections and CD4 counts <350 cells/mm^3. It is also recommended that all pregnant women with any stage 3 disease and CD4 counts <350 cells/mm^3 initiate ART.

In the absence of a CD4 cell count, a TLC <1200 cells/mm^3 in patients with mild symptomatic (WHO stage 2) HIV disease has been recommended as a guide to the initiation of ART. While the TLC correlates relatively poorly with the CD4 cell count in asymptomatic persons, in combination with clinical staging, it has been reported as a useful marker of prognosis and survival.[93]

A fundamental part of initiating treatment is ensuring that the patient is an active and a responsible member of the planning team.

- The key to effective ART and treatment of any comorbidities is a careful assessment and education of the person, leading to the development of an individualized treatment plan to maximize adherence.
- It is crucial that a treatment plan is designed in collaboration with staff, the patient and (where appropriate) the family.
- All predictable potential barriers to successful treatment adherence should be addressed with this plan, although ART may need to be initiated before these barriers can be resolved.
- The active participation of patients in their own treatment encourages closer cooperation with health-care workers and better feedback on the effects of treatment.

5.1. Choice of ART regimen

The basic WHO recommended first- and second-line ARV drug formulary can be used in the regimen selection process for a large majority of patients who inject drugs. However, the high prevalence of comorbidities and cotreatment interactions should be taken into consideration while selecting the preferred drugs. These include the following:

- Comorbidities are very common, in particular, mental health problems such as depression.
- Coinfections such as HCV, HBV and TB are common.
- People who inject drugs may continue to actively use illicit drugs.
- Drug interactions can occur, e.g. interactions between non-nucleoside reverse transcriptase inhibitors (NNRTIs) and methadone.
- People who inject drugs may find it difficult to consistently access ART due to reasons such as homelessness, wanting to avoid law-enforcement authorities, etc.

It is unrealistic and unethical to limit ART to those people who inject drugs and are receiving OST. Therefore, the above considerations have implications for the choice of treatment regimen for people who inject drugs. With the following exceptions, however, the choice of ART should follow treatment guidelines for patients who do not inject drugs.

Specific issues for ART in people who inject drugs include the following:

- Women who wish to become pregnant should **not** be prescribed EFV.
- Active hepatitis may be exacerbated to a greater extent by nevirapine (NVP) than other drugs.
- Hepatotoxicity may be due to direct drug toxicity or a consequence of immune reconstitution inflammatory syndrome (IRIS) in patients with HCV and/or HBV.
- For those who inject drugs and are coinfected with HBV, lamivudine (3TC) and TDF are active against both infections and should be used in the ART regimen, if possible.
- In alcohol users, the potential for pancreatitis and peripheral neuropathy is increased with stavudine (d4T) and didanosine (ddI).
- Intolerance of both NNRTIs due to liver disease (e.g. cirrhosis, chronic hepatitis caused by HCV and HBV), psychiatric disorders or pregnancy may require the use of a triple nucleoside regimen – where abacavir (ABC) or TDF can replace EFV/NVP. (*See* section 5.2 in the WHO 2006 ART guidelines for details.[93])

WHO recommends that the first-line regimen for adults and adolescents contains two nucleoside reverse transcriptase inhibitors (NRTIs) plus one NNRTI (Fig. 1). This recommendation is based on available evidence, clinical experience and programmatic feasibility for the wider introduction of ART in resource-limited settings. Regimens based on a combination of two NRTIs plus one NNRTI are efficacious, generally less expensive than other regimens, have generic formulations, are often available as fixed-dose combinations (FDCs) and do not require a cold chain. In addition, they preserve a potent new class (protease inhibitors [PIs]) for second-line treatment. The disadvantages include different drug half-lives which complicate procedures for stopping ART, the fact that a single mutation is associated with resistance to some drugs (3TC and the NNRTIs), and cross-resistance within the NNRTI class.

The thiacytadine analogues (3TC or emtricitabine [FTC]) are pivotal to first-line regimens. 3TC or FTC should be used with a companion nucleoside or nucleotide analogue, the choices being azidothymidine (AZT), TDF, ABC or d4T. The preferred NRTI backbone is composed of AZT or TDF combined with either 3TC or FTC. ddI is an adenosine analogue NRTI, recommended to be reserved for second-line regimens. Finally, an NNRTI, either EFV or NVP, should be added.

A triple NRTI regimen should be considered as an alternative to first-line ART in situations where NNRTI options provide additional complications, and to preserve the PI class for second-line treatment (e.g. in women with CD4 counts of 250–350 cells/mm³; coinfection with viral hepatitis or TB; severe adverse reactions to NVP and EFV; infection with HIV-2). Recommended triple NRTI combinations are AZT + 3TC + ABC, and AZT + 3TC + TDF (*see* Fig. 1).

Recommended regimens for people who inject drugs are summarized below; however, both the availability of specific ARVs and as well as FDC pills will vary among different countries and regions. Furthermore, this is a rapidly changing field and those prescribing ART should follow regular updates and guidelines.

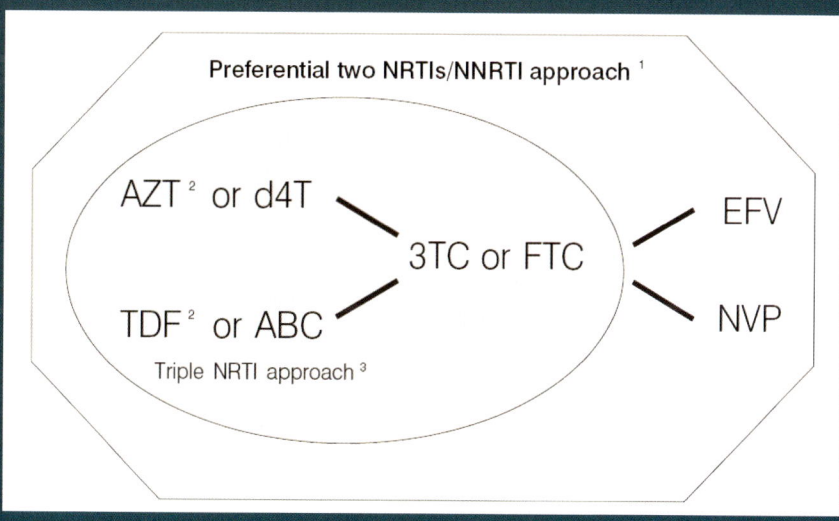

FIG. 1. FIRST-LINE ART REGIMENS FOR ADULTS AND ADOLESCENTS WHO INJECT DRUGS (WHO GUIDELINES 2006[93])

1. The preferential two NRTIs/NNRTI approach is based upon a combination of three drugs: two NRTIs combined with either NVP or EFV as the NNRTI.
2. The preferred NRTI to be combined with 3TC or FTC in standard first-line regimens
3. Triple NRTI approach (three NRTI drugs selected only from the options shown within the circle) can be considered as an alternative to first-line regimens in situations where NNRTI options provide additional complications (e.g. women who have CD4 counts between 250 and 350 cells/mm³, those coinfected with viral hepatitis or TB, severe reactions to NVP or EFV) as discussed above.

Note: The use of ABC and NVP in the same regimen, particularly in people who inject drugs, is probably not a good combination.

TDF/FTC/NNRTI can be a good alternative in HIV/HBV coinfection.

It should be noted that there are important interactions between ARVs and medications commonly used for people who inject drugs (*see* Table 6).

For more details regarding the management of HIV/TB coinfection, please refer to section 10.4 and *Management of collaborative TB/HIV activities: training for managers at the national and subnational levels.*[101]

Switching to second-line ART should be done in case of treatment failure, which is measured clinically and/or immunologically, including by a CD4 cell count.

TABLE 2: RECOMMENDATIONS FOR SWITCHING TO SECOND-LINE ART REGIMENS IN ADULTS

FIRST-LINE REGIMEN		SECOND-LINE REGIMEN	
		RTI COMPONENT	PI COMPONENT [a]
Standard strategy	AZT or d4T + 3TC[b] + NVP or EFV	ddI + ABC or TDF + ABC or TDF + 3TC (+ AZT)[c]	PI/r[d]
	TDF + 3TC[b] + NVP or EFV	ddI + ABC or ddI + 3TC (+ AZT)[c]	
	ABC + 3TC[b] + NVP or EFV	ddI + 3TC (+ AZT)[c] or TDF + 3TC (+ AZT)[c]	
Alternative strategy	AZT or d4T + 3TC[b] + TDF or ABC	EFV or NVP + ddI	

a NFV does not need refrigeration and can be used as a PI alternative in places without a cold chain.
b 3TC and FTC are considered interchangeable because they are structurally related and share pharmacological properties and resistance profiles.
c 3TC can be considered to be maintained in second-line regimens to potentially reduce viral fitness, confer residual antiviral activity and maintain pressure on the *M184V* mutation to improve viral sensitivity to AZT or TDF. AZT may prevent or delay the emergence of the *K65R* mutation.
d There are insufficient data to detect differences among currently available ritonavir (RTV or r)-boosted PIs (ATV/r, FPV/r, IDV/r, LPV/r and saquinavir [SQV]/r) and the choice should be based on individual programme priorities (*see* WHO guidelines 2006[93]). In the absence of a cold chain, NFV can be employed as the PI component but it is considered less potent than an RTV-boosted PI.

Treatment failure (occurrence of a new OI or malignancy, recurrence of a previous OI and the onset of WHO stage 3 conditions) should be differentiated from IRIS, which can occur in the first three months after initiation of ART. IRIS is an inflammatory response to previously subclinical OIs in the setting of advanced immunodeficiency. The OI causing IRIS should be treated as per normal guidelines. In most cases, ART should be discontinued during the initial therapy for the OI responsible for the IRIS. This is discussed further in section 6.1 below.

6. Management of side-effects and toxicity

Side-effects of ARVs are relatively common, reported in nearly 50% of patients, though the majority are mild and self-limiting. Inadequate pre-treatment counselling and poor management of side-effects has led to them to be a leading cause of poor compliance with drug regimens. The need for drug substitution as a result of side-effects occurs in approximately 10–15% of patients commencing ART.[102,103]

Management of possible side-effects is most effective if the patient understands the nature and reasons for the side-effects, and the importance of reporting these early. This is critical for planning and providing adherence support, adjusting treatment regimens so that they are safe, effective and acceptable to the patient, and minimizing the risk of drug resistance because of poor adherence.

Early in the course of ART, mild side-effects such as headache, nausea, diarrhoea and fatigue are common. These may often be managed simply with support, reassurance and symptomatic treatment such as analgesics or antidiarrhoeal agents. These interventions are very useful in helping individuals to cope with side-effects as opposed to stopping or changing their ART regimen.

GUIDING PRINCIPLES IN THE MANAGEMENT OF ARV DRUG TOXICITY

1. Determine the seriousness of the toxicity.

2. Evaluate concurrent medications and establish whether the toxicity is attributable to an ARV drug or drugs or to a non-ARV medication taken at the same time.

3. Consider other disease processes (e.g. viral hepatitis in an individual who develops jaundice while on ARV drugs) because not all problems that arise during treatment are caused by ARV drugs.

4. Manage the adverse event according to the severity. In general:

   - Grade 4 (severe, life-threatening reactions): immediately discontinue all ARV drugs, manage the medical event (i.e. symptomatic and supportive therapy) and reintroduce ARV drugs using a modified regimen (i.e. substituting an ARV for the offending drug) when the patient is stabilized.*

   - Grade 3 (severe reactions): Substitute the offending drug without stopping ART.*

   - Grade 2 (moderate reactions): Consider continuation of ART as long as is feasible. If the patient does not improve on symptomatic therapy, consider single-drug substitution.*

   - Grade 1 (mild reactions): These are bothersome but do not require changes in therapy.

5. Stress the maintenance of adherence despite mild and moderate reactions.

6. If there is a need to discontinue ART because of life-threatening toxicity, all ARV drugs should be stopped until the patient is stabilized.

*See Table 4 for substitution options

Side-effects can vary from mild to very serious and can affect many organ systems. Some examples of major side-effects of ARVs by drug class and organ system are shown in Table 3. Careful clinical assessment is required to exclude other possible causes of signs and symptoms that might be mistaken for side-effects of ARVs; for example, opioid withdrawal syndrome is characterized by headache, anxiety and diarrhoea.[104]

TABLE 3: SIDE-EFFECTS OF ARVs BY DRUG CLASS AND ORGAN SYSTEM[93]

Haematological toxicity	Drug-induced bone marrow suppression, most commonly seen with AZT (anaemia, neutropenia)
Mitochondrial dysfunction	Primarily seen with the NRTI drugs including lactic acidosis, hepatic toxicity, pancreatitis, peripheral neuropathy, lipoatrophy, myopathy
Renal toxicity	Nephrolithiasis, commonly seen with IDV. Renal tubular dysfunction is associated with TDF.
Other metabolic abnormalities	More common with PIs. Include hyperlipidaemia, fat accumulation, insulin resistance, diabetes and osteopenia
Allergic reactions	Skin rashes and hypersensitivity reactions, more common with the NNRTI drugs but also seen with certain NRTI drugs, such as ABC and some PIs

In cases where symptomatic measures are not sufficient or the toxicity is too severe, it will be necessary to substitute one ARV drug with another within the existing ART regimen (Table 4).[93]

TABLE 4: TOXICITIES OF FIRST-LINE ARVs AND RECOMMENDED DRUG SUBSTITUTIONS

ARV DRUG	COMMON ASSOCIATED TOXICITY	SUGGESTED SUBSTITUTE
ABC	Hypersensitivity reaction	AZT or TDF or d4T
AZT	Severe anaemia[a] or neutropenia[b] Severe gastrointestinal intolerance[c]	TDF or d4T or ABC
AZT	Lactic acidosis	TDF or ABC[d]
d4T	Lactic acidosis Lipoatrophy/metabolic syndrome[e]	TDF or ABC[d]
d4T	Peripheral neuropathy	AZT or TDF or ABC
TDF	Renal toxicity (renal tubular dysfunction)	AZT or ABC or d4T
EFV	Persistent and serious central nervous system toxicity[f]	NVP or TDF or ABC (or any PI)[h]
EFV	Potential teratogenicity (first trimester of pregnancy or in women not using adequate contraception)	NVP or ABC (or any PI)[h]
NVP	Hepatitis	EFV or TDF or ABC (or any PI)[h]
NVP	Hypersensitivity reaction	TDF or ABC (or any PI)[h]
NVP	Severe or life-threatening rash (Stevens–Johnson syndrome)[g]	

a Exclude malaria in areas of stable malaria; severe anaemia (grade 4) is defined as Hb <6.5 g/dl.
b Defined as neutrophil cell count <500 cells/mm^3 (grade 4).
c Defined as severe, refractory gastrointestinal intolerance that prevents ingestion of ARV drug regimen (e.g. persistent nausea and vomiting).
d Reinitiation of ART should not include d4T or AZT in this situation. TDF or ABC is preferred.
e Substitution of d4T may not reverse lipoatrophy.
f For example, persistent hallucinations or psychosis
g Severe rash is defined as extensive rash with desquamation, angioedema, or a reaction resembling serum sickness; or a rash with constitutional findings such as fever, oral lesions, blistering, facial oedema or conjunctivitis; Stevens–Johnson syndrome can be life-threatening. For life-threatening rash, substitution with EFV is not recommended, although this approach has been reported in a small number of patients in Thailand without recurrence of rash.
h The PI class should preferentially be reserved for second-line therapy as no potent regimens have been identified for recommendation following initial PI failure.

The substitution of EFV for NVP following a non-severe (grade 1 or 2) NVP-related rash and/or hepatotoxicity is recommended, together with careful monitoring.

6.1. Immune reconstitution inflammatory syndrome (IRIS)

An important and emerging issue with the initiation of ART in individuals with advanced HIV infection is IRIS.[105] This is especially challenging and common in resource-poor settings where ART is not widely available. Table 5 gives an overview of the current state of knowledge on IRIS.

TABLE 5: DESCRIPTION AND MANAGEMENT OF IMMUNE RECONSTITUTION INFLAMMATORY SYNDROME

DEFINITION	A collection of signs and symptoms resulting from the ability to mount an immune response associated with immune recovery on ART[106]
FREQUENCY	10% of all patients initiating ART In up to 25% of patients initiating ART with a CD4 cell count <50 cells/mm^3 [107,108]
TIMING	Typically within 2–12 weeks of initiation of ART but may present later
SIGNS AND SYMPTOMS	Unexpected deterioration of clinical status soon after commencing ART Unmasking of subclinical infections such as TB, which present as new active disease Worsening of coexisting infections such as a flare of hepatitis B or C
MOST COMMON IRIS EVENTS	60% of IRIS events are due to *Mycobacterium tuberculosis*, *Mycobacterium avium* complex (MAC) or cryptococcal disease.[109]
MANAGEMENT	IRIS may be mild and resolve without treatment. Continue ART if the patient can tolerate it. Treat unmasked active OI, such as TB. This may mean temporary interruption of ART until the patient is stable on TB drugs, then reintroduce ART. If the patient is receiving rifampicin and is on NVP, switch to EFV, if available. ABC is a second alternative but EFV is preferred. Switching back to NVP is possible following cessation of therapy with rifampicin. If EFV is not available, continue NVP-based ART. Corticosteroid treatment to suppress exaggerated inflammatory response may be indicated; for example, an acute hepatic flare where viral hepatitis coinfection is known or suspected. If the patient is taking NVP, clinical hepatitis and/or rising hepatic enzymes in association with rash and fever is more likely to be due to NVP than IRIS and switching to EFV is recommended. Prednisone 0.5 mg/kg/day for 5–10 days is suggested in moderate to severe cases of IRIS.[110]

6.2. Hepatotoxicity of antiretroviral (ARV) drugs

Despite the common association between hepatotoxicity and ART, approximately 90% of HIV-infected individuals, regardless of whether they are coinfected with hepatitis viruses, will tolerate ART without severe liver toxicity.[111] Regimens combining d4T and ddI should be avoided because of the increased risk of lactic acidosis and other mitochondrial-related toxicities. Hepatotoxicity has also been associated with the NNRTIs, with NVP being the most likely cause. This is somewhat higher in those with HIV/HCV coinfection but should not preclude the use of NNRTIs. Patients with higher CD4 counts are at higher risk of drug-related hepatitis and monitoring of liver enzymes is recommended.

7. Drug interactions with ARVs

Health-care providers should counsel patients about possible interactions of ARVs with other drugs that they may be taking. This includes OST, illicit or non-prescribed drugs, as well as prescribed medications for medical or psychiatric conditions, OI prophylaxis, OI treatment, HCV and HBV. Being aware of drug interactions and reporting the symptoms of potential interactions in a timely fashion is critical to ensure the safe use of ARVs. In addition, identifying interactions will improve adherence to treatment and ultimately improve effectiveness. The amount and complexity of drug interaction information along with the rapid developments in this area make it extremely challenging for the physician/pharmacist/nurse to keep up to date. In addition to the regularly updated WHO ART guidelines (*see* Annex 5 of the WHO guidelines),[93] helpful websites are available to provide updated information on drug interactions associated with ARVs:

- http://hivinsite.ucsf.edu/arvdb?page=ar-00-02
- http://www.hiv-druginteractions.org

7.1. Substitution medications

7.1.1. Methadone and ARVs

7.1.1.1. Mechanism of interactions between methadone and ARVs

Methadone is metabolized in the liver by several cytochrome P450 enzymes (especially CYP 3A4 enzyme).

7.1.1.2. Management of interactions between other drugs, methadone and ARVs

Opioid metabolism can be inhibited or induced by the concomitant use of PIs or NNRTIs. Patients should be monitored for signs of withdrawal or oversedation and the methadone dose adjusted promptly accordingly. Withdrawal symptoms, if they occur, generally appear within 4–10 days of ART initiation.[112] Withdrawal symptoms should be monitored clinically and the methadone dose increased by 10 mg increments every 3–4 days to effectively manage withdrawal symptoms (the increase in methadone dose may not be as large as expected from pharmacokinetic data).[113] Table 6 gives an overview of the current state of knowledge on the interactions between ARVs and methadone.

TABLE 6: INTERACTIONS BETWEEN ARV DRUGS AND METHADONE

ANTIRETROVIRAL AGENT	EFFECT ON METHADONE	EFFECT OF METHADONE ON ARV AGENT	COMMENT
NRTIs			
Zidovudine (AZT)	None reported	Concentrations increased (up to 43%) and adverse events possible	Monitor for anaemia, myalgia, vomiting, asthenia, headache and bone marrow suppression.
Lamivudine (3TC)	None reported	None reported	No known interactions
Emtricitabine (FTC)	Not studied	Not studied	No known interactions
Tenofovir (TDF)	None reported	None reported	No known interactions
Stavudine (d4T)	None reported	Concentrations decreased (up to 27%)	Clinical significance of effect unclear
Abacavir (ABC)	Methadone levels decreased but dosage adjustments unlikely	Peak concentration reduced (up to 34%)	Data sparse – although one study showed an increase of 22% in oral methadone clearance
Didanosine (ddI) (buffered tablet and enteric-coated [EC] capsule)	None reported. No dosage adjustments necessary	Concentrations decreased (up to 60%) in buffered tablet but not in EC capsule	No effect on EC capsule, therefore preferred
NNRTIs			
Efavirenz (EFV)	Methadone levels decreased (area under the curve [AUC] ↓ up to 60%) and withdrawal symptoms common	Unknown	Monitor and titrate dose if necessary. Increase in methadone dose usually required. Onset of withdrawal symptoms may be delayed up to 3 weeks after starting EFV.
Nevirapine (NVP)	Methadone levels decreased (AUC ↓ up to 46%) and withdrawal symptoms common	None reported	Monitor and titrate dose if necessary. Increase in methadone dose (up to 100%) usually required. Withdrawal symptoms generally occur between 4 and 8 days after starting NVP.
PIs			
Lopinavir/ritonavir (LPV/r)	Methadone levels may be reduced (AUC ↓ up to 53%)	None reported	Monitor and titrate dose if necessary. May require increase in methadone dose
Saquinavir (SQV)	None reported	None reported	Studies limited
Saquinavir 1600 mg /ritonavir 100 mg (SQV/r)	Methadone levels slightly reduced (AUC ↓ up to 20%)	None reported	Monitor and titrate dose if necessary. May require increase in methadone dose
Atazanavir 300 mg/ritonavir 100 mg (ATZ/r)	None reported	None reported	Studies limited
Nelfinavir (NFV)	Methadone levels may be reduced (AUC ↓ up to 47%)	Levels may be reduced but clinical significance unclear	Monitor and titrate dose if necessary. May require increase in methadone dose.

Interactions may occur between medications used to treat comorbidities, including psychiatric disorders, TB and OIs; and ARVs and methadone. Table 7 shows some of these potential drug interactions.

TABLE 7: DRUG INTERACTIONS BETWEEN MEDICATIONS USED BY HIV-POSITIVE PATIENTS ON ARVs AND METHADONE

PSYCHOTROPIC MEDICATIONS	ACTIONS/USES	INTERACTION WITH METHADONE	INTERACTION WITH ARV MEDICATIONS
Alprazolam (benzodiazepine)	Sedative	Additive CNS depression and possible excessive sedation	Alprazolam clearance decreased by up to 41%. Caution with concurrent use of certain benzodiazepines (alprazolam, midazolam and triazolam) and all PIs and EFV
Fluvoxamine (selective serotonin reuptake inhibitor [SSRI])	Treatment of depression and compulsive disorders	Increased methadone levels by up to 26% Associated with cardiac rhythm disturbances, caution when concurrently used with methadone	Not studied or reported

PSYCHOTROPIC HERBAL MEDICATIONS	ACTIONS/USES	INTERACTION WITH METHADONE	INTERACTION WITH ARV MEDICATIONS
St John's wort (*Hypericum perforatum*)	Antidepressant	Possible decrease in methadone levels	IDV level decreased by up to 57%. May lead to decreased response and resistance to NFV

OTHER MEDICATIONS	ACTIONS/USES	INTERACTION WITH METHADONE	INTERACTION WITH ARV MEDICATIONS
Carbamazepine	Anticonvulsant	Possible decrease in methadone levels – may cause withdrawal. Consider using another anticonvulsant as an alternative.	Monitor for toxicities and dose adjustments.
Fluconazole	Antifungal antibiotic	Increased methadone levels (up to 35%). Clinical significance unknown	Potential for bi-directional inhibition between some azole antifungal antibiotics and PIs
Phenobarbital (barbiturate)	Anticonvulsant Sedative	Significant decrease in methadone levels – may cause withdrawal	Consider avoiding concurrent administration of other potent inducers of cytochrome P450 enzymes (e.g. EFV and NVP). The use of barbiturates may also decrease NFV concentrations.
Phenytoin	Anticonvulsant	Significant decrease in methadone levels – may cause withdrawal. Strongly consider using another anticonvulsant as an alternative.	Monitor for toxicities and dose adjustments.
Interferon-alfa + ribavirin (RBV)	Antihepatitis C treatment	Side-effects can mimic opioid withdrawal symptoms	Hepatitis C infection can aggravate the potential hepatotoxicity of several ART regimens.
Rifampicin Rifampicin/isoniazid	Treatment of pulmonary TB	Highly significant decrease in methadone levels (up to 68%) – probable induction of methadone withdrawal. Usually requires increase in methadone dose	PIs generally contraindicated due to unpredictable drug levels. Rifampicin should not be co-administered with LPV, NFV or SQV. Rifabutin may be a potential alternative, but not in combination with SQV.
Sildenafil	Erectile dysfunction agent	Not reported	No effect of sildenafil on PI RTV increases sildenafil level 10-fold and SQV 3-fold

7.1.2. Buprenorphine and ARVs

Interactions between buprenorphine and ARVs are less well researched than those of methadone. The benefits of buprenorphine are similar to those of methadone and may therefore increase adherence and response to ART. In France, where buprenorphine is widely used, studies have shown that patients receiving ART and buprenorphine respond well to treatment.[114]

While in vitro evidence suggests that buprenorphine is metabolized by the cytochrome P450 enzyme (3A4 isomer) and would be affected in a similar manner as methadone by enzyme inducers such as NVP, EFV and RTV, the evidence is not available from clinical trials to support this. To date, limited data exist on the interactions between buprenorphine and ARVs; however, in examining both EFV and AZT the following have been found:

- The co-administration of EFV with buprenorphine lowers buprenorphine levels but does not seem to produce clinical withdrawal.[115]
- AZT administered in conjunction with buprenorphine, unlike methadone, does not lead to an increase in AZT levels.[116]

Supervision of buprenorphine medication can allow directly observed therapy (DOT) with ART, although patients normally do not require buprenorphine doses every day.

7.2. Interactions with illicit or recreational drugs

Interactions between ARVs and psychoactive substances used for non-medical/recreational purposes may have serious clinical consequences in terms of ART efficacy or drug toxicity.[117,118] PIs and NNRTIs can inhibit or induce the cytochrome P450 system in the liver, which is responsible for the metabolism of benzodiazepines, amphetamines and opioids and, as such, clinically important interactions can occur. In addition, the high rate of HCV coinfection in this population leads to liver disease and this is greatly exacerbated by alcohol use and therefore the use of alcohol should be discouraged.

BENZODIAZEPINES

- Those that are primarily dependent on the CYP 3A4 enzyme for metabolism are likely to be affected by the PIs, and those ARVs that cause inhibition of CYP 3A4 may lead to toxicity in terms of drowsiness, confusion and paradoxical aggression.
- The benzodiazepines that are primarily metabolized by CYP 3A4 include midazolam, triazolam, alprazolam and flunitrazepam.
- The benzodiazepines in which CYP 3A4 metabolism plays a minor role include lorazepam, oxazepam, temazepam and diazepam, and no interactions have been reported.

ALCOHOL

- Substantial consumption may reduce ART adherence, alter drug metabolism and increase the risk of drug-induced hepatotoxicity, especially in patients coinfected with HCV.
- Alcohol may enhance the neuropsychiatric changes (sleep disturbances; depression; and behavioural, concentration and personality changes) associated with EFV.
- Of greatest concern is the issue of drug dosing in the presence of hepatic cirrhosis. Given the lack of data on alcohol and ARV drug interactions, caution should be used when prescribing for patients with hepatic impairment.

COCAINE

- Cocaine is metabolized to norcocaine (active hepatotoxic metabolite) primarily by CYP 3A4.
- PIs and other drugs that inhibit CYP 3A4 activity could, in rare instances, lead to cocaine overdose. Special attention must be given to RTV, IDV and EFV, which are potent inhibitors.
- ARVs that induce CYP 3A4 activity, such as NVP, may shift the metabolism of cocaine and create a higher level of the potentially hepatotoxic metabolite.
- Close monitoring is recommended in cases where there is concomitant use of cocaine and ARVs.

AMPHETAMINE, METHAMPHETAMINE AND 3,4 METHYLENEDIOXYMETHAMPHETAMINE (MDMA)

- Amphetamine, methamphetamine and 3,4 methylenedioxymethamphetamine (MDMA) have similar metabolism, mainly through the CYP 2D6 pathway.
- Certain PIs, especially RTV, may cause inhibition of CYP 2D6 and therefore toxicity, potentially leading to overdose.

OPIOID-BASED DRUGS, SUCH AS ILLICIT HEROIN, CODEINE, MORPHINE AND OTHER ANALGESICS

- Interactions with ARVs are similar to those described for methadone.
- NNRTIs and some PIs may result in opioid withdrawal and loss of analgesia.

TETRAHYDROCANNABINOL (THC) (MAIN ACTIVE COMPONENT OF CANNABIS PRODUCTS)

- Limited information in relation to potential interactions with ARVs [119]

OTHER PSYCHOACTIVE DRUGS THAT MAY BE USED NON-MEDICALLY/ RECREATIONALLY

- Gamma-hydroxybutyrate (GBH, Liquid X) toxicity has been reported in a patient taking GBH while on RTV and SQV. [120, 121]
- Phencyclidine might be metabolized primarily by CYP 3A4 and therefore PIs may increase the risk for phencyclidine toxicity.

The lack of research in this area means that some of the interactions or effects are postulated on the basis of knowledge of enzyme substrates involved in the metabolism of various drugs and have not been clinically demonstrated.

8. Adherence

Adherence is the most important determinant of a successful response to ART. High adherence rates (>95%) appear to be required for optimal outcomes in terms of viral suppression.[122] Poor adherence can lead to virological failure, the emergence of drug resistance, and subsequent immunological and clinical failure.[122–124] With the development of drug resistance, there is potential for transmission of drug-resistant virus and the need to revise treatment regimens.[125] The relationship between non-adherence and plasma HIV RNA levels is clear, but not proportionate (i.e. a small amount of non-adherence results in large losses of viral control). One study highlighted that a 10% decrease in adherence was associated with a doubling of the HIV RNA level.[126] In addition to an increase in the HIV RNA levels, the CD4 count can decrease with adherence rates of <90%.[127]

The reported need for >95% adherence to treatment has allowed an incorrect view to develop that people who inject drugs are poor candidates for ART. People who inject drugs have been disproportionately and wrongly excluded from HIV/AIDS treatment. Studies indicate that the proportion of non-adherent individuals is similar between individuals who do not inject drugs, adequately supported people who inject drugs and those who inject drugs and are on OST,[128] and that the rates of ARV resistance are no higher in people who inject drugs than in those who do not.[10]

Active drug use is not a valid criterion for denying people who inject drugs access to care and treatment. People who inject drugs and are engaged in stable care with experienced staff and adequate support can adhere to ART and have clinical outcomes equivalent to those of HIV-infected patients who do not use drugs.[10,129] In particular, consistent participation in a methadone maintenance treatment programme has been shown to be associated with a higher probability of ART use and, among these, a more consistent adherence to ART.[130,131,132]

8.1. Factors influencing adherence

One of the most important aspects of optimizing adherence is patient education. In many Asian settings, experience with chronic therapies would be limited and patient information is critical. In China, it was recently shown that knowledge about ART among HIV-positive people who inject drugs was extremely limited.[133] Adherence to ART or lack of it can be influenced by many factors including:

- toxicity and side-effects of ARV drugs or interactions with other medications, including OST and alcohol;
- hepatitis, which occurs more often among people who inject drugs and should be closely monitored;
- OIs including IRIS
- comorbid psychiatric disorders, including depression;
- depression, which is also a determinant of clinical progression independent of adherence;[134,135]
- continuing drug use or relapse;
- the lack of future prospects and motivation, which may be linked to a range of social problems including unemployment, homelessness and family issues;
- perceived side-effects of ARVs;[136]
- expectations of treatment success;
- stigma and discrimination in health-care settings and providers who not believe that people who inject drugs can adequately adhere to ART;[137,138]
- unfriendly and poor quality of health services according to the patient's perception;
- availability and accessibility of treatment services for drug dependence; and
- restrictive legislative and policy issues.

8.2. Adherence support

Optimizing adherence in the early months (4–6 months) of treatment is crucial to ensure long-term success.[139] Moderate deviations from high adherence (88–99%) during follow up (maintenance phase after 6 months) have less of a negative impact. Several interventions for enhancing adherence are possible, but priority should be given to interventions aimed at improving adherence in the early months of ART.[140–142] Adherence support should be part of the routine clinical care provided by all health professionals involved in dealing with HIV-infected individuals. Staff should provide individualized support for adherence based on the needs of each patient at any given time in their treatment.

8.2.1. Patient counselling

While counselling patients on adherence, health-care providers should also consider a range of other issues, including whether the patient:

- has emotional and practical life-supports;
- can fit his/her ART regimen into a daily routine;
- understands that non-adherence leads to resistance and treatment failure;
- recognizes that all doses must be taken;
- feels comfortable taking ARVs in front of others;
- keeps clinical appointments; and
- understands the interactions and side-effects of ARVs taken in combination with OST and illicit drugs.

8.2.2. Other strategies

There are a number of other strategies that can be helpful in optimizing adherence:

- Provide practical aids to enhancing adherence, including travel/transportation support, use of family/friends/peers to help in attending appointments and supporting daily ART use.
- Maintain a system for tracking/outreach that can accurately and rapidly find those who have been lost to follow up. Home visits can be useful if the patient's status is known by family members. It is essential to minimize stigma through psychosocial support.
- Family or community members should be engaged in adherence education and maintenance programmes. Family-based care is desirable if more than one family member is HIV-infected, particularly when mother and child are infected.
- Manage drug interactions and adjust drug doses in a timely fashion.
- Dispense medication in small amounts at frequent intervals as this can lead to:
  - opportunities to detect and address adherence problems before they lead to drug resistance; and
  - limited disruptions in or misuse of treatment. Pillboxes or coblister packs can be used.
- Provide medications free of charge for people who can least afford treatment through subsidized or other financing strategies. Free access to ARVs at the point of delivery may assist adherence.
- Adopt DOT or modified DOT strategies. This approach is resource-intensive and difficult to introduce on a large scale and for the lifelong duration of ART. However, it may be helpful for certain groups (people who inject drugs) and for early patient training.
- Develop strategies for reaching isolated communities.
- In the early stage of treatment, try to provide once-daily options and a low pill burden. The use of FDCs may be of benefit.

9. Management principles of acute and chronic pain relief (including for people on OST)

Pain management in opioid-dependent individuals is unnecessarily controversial. Clinicians may be reluctant to prescribe adequate pain relief drugs, resulting in patients sourcing their own drugs, perhaps illicitly. Patients do not obtain adequate pain relief from their usual daily dose of methadone. Additional analgesics should be prescribed to treat acute or chronic pain in HIV-infected people who inject drugs, whether or not they are on OST. The following factors should be considered:

- Methadone given in a daily dose for the treatment of opioid dependence is not effective in treating pain and therefore methadone-maintained individuals need additional interventions to control pain.
- Consider alternative options for pain relief, e.g. acupuncture, massage, particularly in situations of chronic pain.
- Careful monitoring is required when people who inject drugs and are on ART need ongoing pain relief medication, as dose adjustments or a change in the timing of administration may be necessary.
- Clinicians should treat pain in people who inject drugs and are maintained on methadone in the same way that they would in non-methadone maintained individuals.
- Patients who are maintained on methadone have tolerance to opioids and may need higher-than-expected doses of opioids for analgesic action.

Further clinical studies are needed of patients being treated for pain while receiving buprenorphine. As with methadone, buprenorphine does have analgesic properties; however, the once-daily dose for the treatment of substance use may not be sufficient to sustain pain relief. Opioid analgesia may be minimally effective in patients maintained on buprenorphine because of its pharmacokinetic properties. Nonetheless, patients require effective pain management. As such:

- Patients receiving buprenorphine and in need of pain relief should first be treated with a non-opioid analgesic when appropriate.
- A temporary increase in buprenorphine dose may provide the additional analgesia needed.
- If there is acute pain that is not relieved by non-opioid medications or an increase in the dose of buprenorphine, more aggressive treatment should be given.
- When patients being treated with buprenorphine require other opioid treatment for pain, the following should be borne in mind:
  - Avoid morphine in patients maintained on buprenorphine.
  - While taking other opioid pain medication, buprenorphine should be discontinued.
  - Higher doses of short-acting opioid pain medication may be needed to achieve analgesia until the buprenorphine is cleared from the body.
  - Once the body is cleared of buprenorphine, the dosage of pain medication should be decreased.
  - Buprenorphine should not be restarted until an appropriate period after the last dose of the opioid analgesic; this is dependent on the half-life of the opioid analgesic used.
  - Non-combination opioid analgesics are preferred to avoid toxicity, other side-effects and for easier dosing.
  - Patients with chronic pain who do not respond to increased buprenorphine and require ongoing additional analgesia may need to be transferred to methadone treatment.[142]

10. Coinfections and comorbidities with HIV in people who inject drugs

10.1. Hepatitis B (HBV)

HBV and HIV share similar routes of transmission and are found in the same endemic areas. However, HBV is about 100 times more infectious than HIV. Consequently, more than 70% of HIV-infected people have a blood marker of past or present HBV infection. Men who have sex with men (MSM) have higher rates of HBV/HIV coinfection than people who inject drugs. ART for patients with HBV coinfection should preferentially include 3TC and TDF, as both the drugs have activity against HIV and HBV.

10.2. Hepatitis C (HCV)

The rate of HCV coinfection in HIV-infected people who inject drugs is between 60% and 90%.[143–145] Despite the fact that spontaneous viral clearance may occur in up to 25% of patients or even higher in some studies,[146] there remains a chance of re-infection and ongoing chronic liver disease.[147]

The side-effects of hepatitis treatment have the potential to destabilize a successful response to ART. Consideration should be given to the administration of anti-HCV therapy at the substance dependence centre or HIV/AIDS centre where OST and ART may be directly administered. A further advantage of this approach is that the patient can be monitored clinically by the psychiatric/psychological supports in the drug dependence service, as depression is one of the more serious side-effects of interferon therapy.[148]

HCV-positive patients should be considered for therapy with pegylated interferon and RBV. The sustained response rate for treatment with pegylated interferon and RBV has been found to be between 11% and 29% for genotype 1, and 43–73% in infection with non-type 1 genotypes.[149–151] This modest response to treatment means that serious consideration is required before patients are started on this therapy. Factors influencing response include the CD4 count, HIV viral load and presence/absence of cirrhosis. Treatment is best provided at a high CD4 count before the need for ART arises. If the patient does require intervention with ART, this should be given and the patient stabilized on therapy with a CD4 count of >200 cells/mm^3 before anti-HCV treatment is initiated.

10.3. Chronic liver disease

Concurrent infections with HBV and HCV are a growing cause for concern as they can lead to cirrhosis and hepatocellular carcinoma. HBV and HCV are much more common in HIV-infected individuals than in the population as a whole. Chronic liver disease resulting from these infections progresses more rapidly in HIV-infected patients, increasing mortality rates in this group. Alcohol-related liver disease is also prevalent in people who inject drugs.

10.4. Active tuberculosis (TB) and HIV/TB in people who inject drugs

The treatment of TB and HIV coinfection in all patients is complex; however, it can still be managed effectively.[152,153] Data supporting specific treatment recommendations are incomplete and further research is needed in this area. The availability of antituberculosis medications and the regional patterns of resistant TB must be considered.

In the presence of TB, rifampicin should not be administered to patients receiving PIs (risk of developing possible drug-induced hepatitis). Table 8 suggests some of the most appropriate regimens for treatment of the coinfection.

TABLE 8: ART RECOMMENDATIONS FOR PATIENTS WHO DEVELOP TB WITHIN SIX MONTHS OF STARTING A FIRST-LINE OR SECOND-LINE ART REGIMEN[93]

FIRST-LINE OR SECOND-LINE ART	ART REGIMEN AT THE TIME TB OCCURS	OPTIONS
First-line ART	Two NRTIs + EFV	Continue with two NRTIs + EFV
	Two NRTIs + NVP	• Substitute with EFV[ab] or • Change to triple NRTI regimen[a] or • Continue with two NRTIs + NVP[c]
	Triple NRTI regimen	Continue triple NRTI regimen
Second-line ART	Two NRTIs + PI	Substitute with or continue (if already being taken) LPV/r- or SQV/r-containing regimen and adjust dose of RTV[a]

a Substituting back to the original regimens once the rifampicin-containing regimen is completed can be considered. When switching back from EFV to NVP, no lead-in dose is required.
b The use of EFV-containing regimens is not recommended in women with childbearing potential if adequate contraception cannot be ensured and during the first trimester of pregnancy.
c Careful clinical and laboratory monitoring (ALT) is advised when NVP or boosted PIs are administered concurrently with rifampicin.

The dose of methadone needs to be considered while treating TB in people who inject drugs. As rifampicin is a potent inducer of cytochrome P450, this can lead to a reduction in circulating methadone levels, requiring an increase in the methadone dose. Buprenorphine is also metabolized by the cytochrome P450 pathway and prescribing rifampicin may have an impact on the dose of buprenorphine.

10.5. Other coinfections and comorbidities

Other comorbidities that occur more frequently among people who inject drugs include:
- deep venous thrombosis (DVT) and pulmonary embolism;
- increased risk of respiratory and other smoking-related illnesses, and chronic diseases; and
- bacterial infections as a consequence of IDU and a striking feature of HIV disease. The following conditions occur frequently among people who inject drugs:
  - skin infection and soft tissue abscesses;
  - bacterial pneumonia, which tends to be an earlier and more common manifestation in such patients (CD4 count 200–400 cells/mm^3)[154] ; and
  - endocarditis and septicaemia.

10.6. Prevention and support for treatment of coinfections and comorbidities

Management of comorbidities can have a significant impact on the treatment outcome of HIV-infected people who inject drugs. As many of the comorbidities can be managed through active prevention programmes, treatment services should consider the following points:

- Provide information on injecting techniques to decrease the complications of injection, such as soft tissue and vascular damage and infection.
- Diagnose and treat mental health problems.
- Provide prophylaxis/suppression for specific HIV-related OIs as needed (e.g. *Pneumocystis jiroveci* pneumonia [PCP], candidiasis, cryptococcosis, toxoplasmosis, MAC, cytomegalovirus [CMV]).
- Offer vaccination for HBV to those not vaccinated or not already infected.
- Provide palliative care for patients with advanced disease.

References

1. WHO, UNAIDS and UNODC. *Evidence for action on HIV/AIDS and injecting drug use. Policy brief: antiretroviral therapy and injecting drug users.* Geneva, WHO, 2005 (WHO/HIV/2005.06).

2. Aceijas C et al. Antiretroviral treatment for injecting drug users in developing and transitional countries one year before the end of the "Treating 3 million by 2005. Making it happen. The WHO strategy" ('3by5'). *Addiction*, 2006, 101:1246–1253.

3. Open Society Institute. *Breaking down barriers. Lessons on providing HIV treatment to IDUs.* New York, International Harm Reduction Development (IHRD), Open Society Institute, 2004.

4. Open Society Institute. *Protecting the rights of injection drug users. The impact of HIV and AIDS.* New York, International Harm Reduction Development (IHRD), Open Society Institute, 2004.

5. Kohli R et al. Mortality in an urban cohort of HIV-infected and at-risk drug users in the era of highly active antiretroviral therapy. *Clinical Infectious Diseases*, 2005, 41:864–872.

6. Celentano DD et al. Time to initiating highly active antiretroviral therapy among HIV-infected injection drug users. *AIDS*, 2001, 15:1707–1715.

7. Van Asten LC et al. Limited effect of highly active antiretroviral therapy among HIV-positive injecting drug users on the population level. *European Journal of Public Health*, 2003, 13:347–349.

8. Wood E et al. Extending access to HIV antiretroviral therapy to marginalised populations in the developed world. *AIDS*, 2003, 17:2419–2427.

9. Wood E et al. Adherence and plasma HIV RNA responses to highly active antiretroviral therapy among HIV-1 infected injection drug users. *Canadian Medical Association Journal*, 2003, 169:656–661.

10. Wood E et al. Rates of antiretroviral resistance among HIV-infected patients with and without a history of injection drug use. *AIDS*, 2005, 19:1189–1195.

11. Clarke S et al. Directly observed antiretroviral therapy for injection users with HIV infection. *AIDS Reader*, 2003, 12:312–316.

12. Mesquita F. Brazil: giving IDUs access to HAART as a response to the HIV/AIDS epidemic. In: Open Society Institute. *Breaking down barriers. Lessons on providing HIV treatment to IDUs.* New York, International Harm Reduction Development (IHRD), Open Society Institute, 2004.

13. Sambamoorthi U et al. Drug abuse, methadone treatment and health services use among injection drug users with AIDS. *Drug and Alcohol Dependence*, 2000, 60:77–89.

14. Aceijas C et al. Global overview of injecting drug use and HIV infection among injecting drug users. *AIDS*, 2004, 18:2295–2303.

15. *Joint UNAIDS statement on HIV prevention and care strategies for drug users.* Geneva, UNAIDS, 2005.
http://www.unaids.org/html/pub/una-docs/cco_idupolicy_en_pdf.htm

16. Eicher AD et al. A certain fate: spread of HIV among young injecting drug users in Manipur, north-east India. *AIDS Care*, 2000, 12:497–504.

17. Ministry of Health of Indonesia. *Report on HIV/AIDS cases to March of 2006.* Jakarta, Ministry of Health, 2006.

18. Tang YL et al. Opiate addiction in China: current situation and treatments. *Addiction*, 2006, 101: 657–665.

19. Khoshnood K et al. Assessing the feasibility of introducing voluntary counseling and testing (VCT) in mandatory detoxification and re-education centers for injecting drug users (IDUs) and commercial sex workers (CSW) in China. Presented at the XVI International AIDS Conference, Toronto, Canada, 13–18 August 2006. Abstract TUPE0384.

20. Haberer J et al. A model of care providing antiretroviral therapy to Chinese intravenous drug users with HIV/AIDS. Presented at the XVI International AIDS Conference, Toronto, Canada, 13–18 August 2006. Abstract CDB1032.

21. Riono P, Jazant S. The current situation of the HIV/AIDS epidemic in Indonesia. *AIDS Education and Prevention*, 2004, 16(3 Suppl A):78–90.

22. Nguyen TH, Nguyen TL, Trinh QH. HIV/AIDS epidemics in Vietnam: evolution and responses. *AIDS Education and Prevention*, 2004, 16 (3 Suppl A):137–154.

23. Grassly NC et al. Modelling emerging HIV epidemics: the role of injecting drug use and sexual transmission in the Russian Federation, China and India. *International Journal of Drug Policy*, 2003, 14: 5–43.

24. Shakarishvili A et al. Sex work, drug use, HIV infection, and spread of sexually transmitted infections in Moscow, Russian Federation. *Lancet*, 2005, 366:57–60.

25. Xiao Y et al. Expansion of HIV/AIDS in China: lessons from Yunnan Province. *Social Science and Medicine*, 2007, 64:665–675.

26. Sarkar K et al. Epidemic of HIV coupled with hepatitis C virus among injecting drug users of Himalayan West Bengal, Eastern India, bordering Nepal, Bhutan, and Bangladesh. *Substance Use and Misuse*, 2006, 41:341–352.

27. Go V et al. High HIV sexual risk behaviors and sexually transmitted disease prevalence among injection drug users in Northern Vietnam: implications for a generalized HIV epidemic. *Journal of Acquired Immune Deficiency Syndromes*, 2006, 42:108–115.

28. Panda S et al. Risk factors for HIV infection in injection drug users and evidence for onward transmission of HIV in their sexual partners in Chennai, India. *Journal of Acquired Immune Deficiency Syndromes*, 2005, 39:9–15.

29. Choi SY, Cheung YW, Chen K. Gender and HIV risk behavior among intravenous drug users in Sichuan Province, China. *Social Science and Medicine*, 2006, 62:1672–1684.

30. Kassutto S, Rosenberg ES. Primary HIV type 1 infection. *Clinical Infectious Diseases*, 2004, 38:1447–1453.

31. WHO, UNDOC and UNAIDS. *Position paper: substitution maintenance therapy in the management of opioid dependence and HIV/AIDS prevention.* Geneva, WHO, 2004a
   http://whqlibdoc.who.int/unaids/2004/9241591153.pdf

32. Potvin S, Sepehry AA, Stip E. A meta-analysis of negative symptoms in dual diagnosis schizophrenia. *Psychological Medicine*, 2006, 36:431–440.

33. Green AI, Brown ES. Comorbid schizophrenia and substance abuse. *Journal of Clinical Psychiatry*, 2006, 67:e08.

34. Regier D et al. Comorbidity of mental disorders with alcohol and other drug abuse: results from the Epidemiologic Catchment Area (ECA) study. *Journal of the American Medical Association*, 1990, 264:2511–2518.

35. Bouhnik AD et al. Non-adherence among HIV-infected injecting drug users: the impact of social instability. *Journal of Acquired Immune Deficiency Syndromes*, 2002, 31 (Suppl 3):S149–S153.

36. Bouhnik AD et al. Depression and clinical progression in HIV-infected drug users treated with highly active antiretroviral therapy. *Antiviral Therapy*, 2005, 10:53–61.

37. Paxton S et. al. AIDS-related discrimination in Asia. *AIDS Care*, 2005, 2:145–151.

38. Buavirat A et al. Risk of prevalent HIV infection associated with incarceration among injecting drug users in Bangkok, Thailand: case–control study. *British Medical Journal*, 2003, 326:308.

39. *Status paper on prisons, drugs and harm reduction.* Copenhagen, World Health Organization Regional Office for Europe, 2005.

40. UNODC. *HIV/AIDS prevention, care, treatment and support in prison settings – a framework for an effective national response.* October 2006.
   http://www.undoc.org/unodc/en/drug_demand_hiv_aids_policy.html

41. Altice FL et al. Developing a directly administered antiretroviral therapy intervention for HIV-infected drug users: implications for program replication. *Clinical Infectious Diseases*, 2004, 38 (Suppl 5):S376–S387.

42. Inungu J, Beach EM, Skeel R. Challenges facing health professionals caring for HIV-infected drug users. *AIDS Patient Care and STDs,* 2003, 17:333–343.

43. Des Jarlais DC, Semaan S. Interventions to reduce the sexual risk behaviour of injecting drug users. *International Journal of Drug Policy (Suppl)*, 2005, 16S:S58–S66.

44. Farrell M et al. Effectiveness of drug dependence treatment in HIV prevention. *International Journal of Drug Policy (Suppl)*, 2005, 16S:S67–S75.

45. Wodak A, Cooney A. Effectiveness of sterile needle and syringe programmes. *International Journal of Drug Policy (Suppl)*, 2005, 16S:S31–S44.

46. *Evidence for action technical paper: effectiveness of sterile needle and syringe programming in reducing HIV/AIDS among injecting drug users.* Geneva, World Health Organization, 2004b.
http://www.who.int/hiv/pub/prev_care/en/effectivenesssterileneedle.pdf

47. *Evidence for action technical paper: effectiveness of community-based outreach in preventing HIV/AIDS among injecting drug users.* Geneva, World Health Organization, 2004c.
http://www.who.int/hiv/pub/prev_care/en/evidenceforactionreprint2004.pdf

48. *Evidence for action technical paper: Effectiveness of drug dependence treatment in preventing HIV among injecting drug users.* Geneva, World Health Organization, 2004d.
http://www.who.int/hiv/pub/idu/en/drugdependencefinaldraft.pdf

49. WHO, UNDOC and UNAIDS. *Evidence for action on HIV/AIDS and injecting drug use. Policy brief: provision of sterile injecting equipment to reduce HIV transmission.* Geneva, World Health Organization, 2004b (WHO/HIV/2004.03).
http://www.who.int/hiv/pub/advocacy/en/provisionofsterileen.pdf

50. WHO, UNDOC and UNAIDS. *Evidence for action on HIV/AIDS and injecting drug use. Policy brief: reduction of HIV transmission through drug-dependence treatment.* Geneva, World Health Organization, 2004c (WHO/HIV/2004.04).
http://www.who.int/hiv/pub/advocacy/en/drugdependencetreatmenten.pdf

51. WHO, UNDOC and UNAIDS. *Evidence for action on HIV/AIDS and injecting drug use. Policy brief: reduction of HIV transmission in prisons.* Geneva, World Health Organization, 2004d (WHO/HIV/2004.05).
http://www.who.int/hiv/pub/advocacy/en/transmissionprisonen.pdf

52. WHO, UNDOC and UNAIDS. *Evidence for action on HIV/AIDS and injecting drug use. Policy brief: reduction of HIV transmission through outreach.* Geneva, World Health Organization, 2004e (WHO/HIV/2004.02).
http://www.who.int/hiv/pub/advocacy/en/throughoutreachen.pdf

53. WHO, UNDOC and UNAIDS. *Evidence for action on HIV/AIDS and injecting drug use. Policy brief: antiretroviral therapy and injection drug users.* Geneva, World Health Organization, 2005 (WHO/HIV/2005.06).
http://www.who.int/hiv/pub/prev_care/arvidu.pdf

54. Chen Y et al. Outreach-based needle and syringe exchange among injecting drug users in China's Hunan province. Presented at the XVI International AIDS Conference, Toronto, Canada, 13–18 August 2006. Abstract TUPE0564.

55. Mesquita F et al. Public health: the leading force of the Indonesian response to HIV/AIDS crises among people who inject drugs. *Harm Reduction Journal*, 2007, 4:9.

56. Mattick RP et al. Methadone maintenance therapy versus no opioid replacement therapy for opioid dependence (Cochrane review). In: *The Cochrane Library*, 2002, Issue 4.

57. Farrell M et al. Methadone maintenance treatment in opiate dependence: a review. *British Medical Journal*, 1994, 309:997–1001.

58. Johnson BA. Pills for speedballing and cocaine dependence. *Lancet*, 2006, 367:1714–1716.

59. Mattick R, Hall W. Are detoxification programmes effective? *Lancet*, 1996, 347:97–100.

60. Lucas GM et al. Directly administered antiretroviral therapy in an urban methadone maintenance clinic: a nonrandomized comparative study. *Clinical Infectious Diseases*, 2004, 38 (Suppl 5):S409–S413.

61. Kerr T et al. Psychosocial determinants of adherence to highly active antiretroviral therapy among injection drug users in Vancouver. *Antiviral Therapy*, 2004, 16:407–414.

62. Wohl DA, Rosen D, Kaplan AH. HIV and incarceration: dual epidemics. *AIDS Reader*, 2006, 16:247–250, 257–260.

63. Kirkland LR et al. Response to lamivudine–zidovudine plus abacavir twice daily in antiretroviral-naive, incarcerated patients with HIV infection taking directly observed treatment. *Clinical Infectious Diseases*, 2002, 34:511–518.

64. Springer SA et al. Effectiveness of antiretroviral therapy among HIV-infected prisoners: reincarceration and the lack of sustained benefit after release to the community. *Clinical Infectious Diseases*, 2004, 38:1754–1760.

65. Lines R et al. *Prison needle exchange: a review of international evidence and experience*. Montreal, Canadian HIV/AIDS Legal Network, 2004. Available at www.aidslaw.ca (cited 8 December 2004).

66. Stöver H, Hennebel LC, Casselman J. *Substitution treatment in European prisons. A study of policies and practices of substitution in prisons in 18 European countries*. London, Cranstoun Drug Services Publishing, 2004.

67. Miller P, Sawa S. Indonesia sets up prison methadone maintenance treatment; news and notes. *Addiction*, 2006, 101:1525–1527.

68. Palepu A et al. Factors associated with the response to antiretroviral therapy among HIV-infected patients with and without a history of injection drug use. *AIDS*, 2001, 15:423–424.

69. Meade CS, Sikkema KJ. HIV risk among adults with severe mental illness: a systematic review. *Clinical Psychology Review*, 2005, 25:433–457.

70. Bruce RD, Altice FL. Editorial comment: Why treat three conditions when it is one patient? *AIDS Reader*, 2003, 13:378–379.

71. Yun L et al. Antidepressant treatment improves adherence to antiretroviral therapy among depressed HIV-infected patients. *Journal of Acquired Immune Deficiency Syndromes*, 2005, 38:432–438.

72. Johnson RE et al. A comparison of levomethadyl acetate, buprenorphine and methadone for opioid dependence. *New England Journal of Medicine*, 2000, 343: 1290–1297.

73. Pang L et al. Progress of China's methadone maintenance treatment programme. Presented at the XVI International AIDS Conference, Toronto, Canada, 13–18 August 2006. Abstract TUPDB01.

74. *Proposal for the inclusion of methadone in the WHO Model List of Essential Medicines*. Geneva, World Health Organization Department of Mental Health, 2004e.

75. Auriacombe M et al. French field experience with buprenorphine. *American Journal on Addictions*, 2004, 13 (Suppl 1):S17–S28.

76. Jenkinson RA et al. Buprenorphine diversion and injection in Melbourne, Australia: an emerging issue? *Addiction*, 2005, 100:197–205.

77. O'Connor J et al. Buprenorphine abuse among opiate addicts. *British Journal of Addiction*, 1988, 83:1085–1087.

78. *Proposal for the inclusion of buprenorphine in the WHO Model List of Essential Medicines*. Geneva, World Health Organization Department of Mental Health and Substance Abuse, 2004f.

79. Celentano DD et al. Self reported antiretroviral therapy in injection drug users. *Journal of the American Medical Association*, 1998, 280:544–546.

80. Rehm J et al. Feasibility, safety, and efficacy of injectable heroin prescription for refractory opioid addicts: a follow-up study. *Lancet*, 2001, 358:1417–1420.

81. Baker A et al. Brief cognitive behavioural interventions for regular amphetamine users: a step in the right direction. *Addiction*, 2005, 100:367–378.

82. Higgins ST et al. Contingent reinforcement increases cocaine abstinence during outpatient treatment and 1 year of follow-up. *Journal of Consulting and Clinical Psychology*, 2000, 68:64–72.

83. Rawson RA et al. A comparison of contingency management and cognitive–behavioural approaches for stimulant-dependent individuals. *Addiction*, 2006, 101:267–274.

84. Rawson RA et al. A multi-site comparison of psychosocial approaches for the treatment of methamphetamine dependence. *Addiction*, 2004, 99:708–717.

85. Vongsheree S et al. High HIV-1 prevalence among methamphetamine users in central Thailand, 1999–2000. *Journal of the Medical Association of Thailand*, 2001, 84:1263–1267.

86. Tyndall MW et al. Intensive injection cocaine use a primary risk factor in the Vancouver HIV-1 epidemic. *AIDS*, 2003, 17:911–913..

87. Beyrer C et al. Methamphetamine users in northern Thailand: changing demographics and risks for HIV and STD among treatment-seeking substance abusers. *International Journal of STD and AIDS*, 2004, 15:697–704.

88. Shearer J et al. Substitution therapy for amphetamine users. *Drug and Alcohol Review*, 2002, 21:179–185.

89. Kampman KM et al. Effectiveness of propranolol for cocaine dependence may depend on cocaine withdrawal symptom severity. *Drug and Alcohol Dependence*, 2001, 63:69–78.

90. Ghodse H. *Drugs and addictive behaviour*. 3rd edition. Oxford, Blackwell Science, 2002.

91. Kampman KM et al. A pilot trial of topiramate for the treatment of cocaine dependence. *Drug and Alcohol Dependence*, 2004, 75:233–240.

92. McCance-Katz EF, Kosten TR, Jatlow P. Disulfiram effects on acute cocaine administration. *Drug and Alcohol Dependence*, 1998, 52:27–39.

93. *Antiretroviral therapy for HIV infection in adults and adolescents in resource-limited settings: towards universal access. Recommendations for a public health approach.* Geneva, World Health Organization, 2006. http://www.who.int/hiv/pub/guidelines/WHO%20Adult%20ART%20Guidelines.pdf http://www.who.int/entity/hiv/art/ARTadultsaddendum.pdf

94. *WHO consultation on technical and operational recommendations for scale-up of laboratory services and monitoring HIV antiretroviral therapy in resource-limited settings.* Geneva, World Health Organization, 2005. http://www.who.int/entity/hiv/pub/meetingreports/labmeetingreport.pdf

95. Egger M et al. Prognosis of HIV1-infected patients starting highly active antiretroviral therapy: a collaborative analysis of prospective studies. *Lancet*, 2002, 360:119–129.

96. Gulick RM et al. Treatment with indinavir, zidovudine, and lamivudine in adults with human immunodeficiency virus infection and prior antiretroviral therapy. *New England Journal of Medicine*, 1997, 337:734–739.

97. Hammer SM et al. A controlled trial of two nucleoside analogues plus indinavir in persons with human immunodeficiency virus infection and CD4 cell counts of 200 per cubic millimeter or less. *New England Journal of Medicine*, 1997, 337:725–733.

98. Garcia F et al. Long-term CD4+ T-cell response to highly active antiretroviral therapy according to baseline CD4+ T-cell count. *Journal of Acquired Immune Deficiency Syndromes*, 2004, 36:702–713.

99. Teerawattananon Y et al. Targeting antiretroviral therapy: lessons from a longitudinal study of morbidity and treatment in relation to CD4 count in Thailand. *Asia-Pacific Journal of Public Health*, 2006, 18:39–48.

100. Wood E et al. When to initiate antiretroviral therapy in HIV-1 infected adults: a review for clinicians and patients. *Lancet Infectious Diseases*, 2005, 5:407–414.

101. *Management of collaborative TB/HIV activities: training for managers at the national and subnational levels.* Geneva, World Health Organization, 2005 (WHO/HTM/TB/2005.359a,b,c).
http://www.who.int/tb/publications/who_htm_tb_2005_359/en/index.html

102. Fellay J et al. Prevalence of adverse events associated with potent antiretroviral treatment: Swiss HIV cohort study. *Lancet*, 2001, 358:1322–1327.

103. Dielemann JP et al. Determinants of recurrent toxicity-driven switches of highly active antiretroviral therapy. *AIDS*, 2002, 16:737–745.

104. Schiller DS. Identification, management and prevention of adverse effects associated with highly active antiretroviral therapy. *American Journal of Health-System Pharmacists*, 2004, 61:2507–2522.

105. Bonnet MM et al. Tuberculosis after HAART initiation in HIV-positive patients from five countries with a high tuberculosis burden. *AIDS*, 2006, 20:1275–1279.

106. Robertson J et al. Immune reconstitution syndrome in HIV: validating a case definition and identifying clinical predictors in persons initiating antiretroviral therapy. *Clinical Infectious Diseases*, 2006, 42:1639–1646.

107. French MA et al. Immune restoration disease after the treatment of immunodeficient HIV-infected patients with highly active antiretroviral therapy. *HIV Medicine*, 2000, 1:107–115.

108. Breen RAM et al. Paradoxical reactions during tuberculosis treatment in patients with and without HIV coinfection. *Thorax*, 2004, 59:704–707.

109. Lipman M, Breen R. Immune reconstitution inflammatory syndrome in HIV. *Current Opinion in Infectious Diseases*, 2006, 19:20–25.

110. McComsey G et al. Placebo-controlled trial of prednisone in advanced HIV-1 infection. *AIDS*, 2001, 15:321–327.

111. Sulkowski MS et al. Hepatotoxicity associated with antiretroviral therapy in adults infected with the human immunodeficiency virus and the role of hepatitis C or B virus infection. *Journal of the American Medical Association*, 2000, 283:74–80.

112. McCance-Katz EF et al. The protease inhibitor lopinavir/ritonavir may produce opiate withdrawal in methadone-maintained patients. *Clinical Infectious Diseases*, 2003, 37:476–482.

113. Altice F, Friedland G, Cooney E. Nevirapine induced opiate withdrawal among injection drug users with HIV receiving methadone. *AIDS*, 1999, 13:957–962.

114. Carrieri MP et al. The Manif-2000 Study Group. Evaluation of buprenorphine maintenance treatment in a French cohort of HIV-infected injecting drug users. *Drug and Alcohol Dependence*, 2003, 72:13–21.

115. McCance-Katz EF et al. Efavirenz decreases buprenorphine exposure, but is not associated with opiate withdrawal in opioid dependent individuals. 12th Conference on Retroviruses and Opportunistic Infections (Program and Abstracts), Boston, Mass, United States, 22–25 February 2005. Abstract 653.

116. McCance-Katz EF et al. Effect of opioid dependence pharmacotherapies on zidovudine disposition. *American Journal on Addictions*, 2001, 10:296–307.

117. Antoniou T, Tseng L. Interactions between recreational drugs and antiretroviral agents. *The Annals of Pharmacotherapy*, 2002, 36:1598–1613.

118. Wynn GH et al. Med–psych drug–drug interactions update. Antiretrovirals, part III: antiretrovirals and drugs of abuse. *Psychosomatics*, 2005, 46:79–87.

119. Kosel BW et al. The effects of cannabinoids on pharmacokinetics of indinavir and nelfinavir. *AIDS*, 2002, 16:534–550.

120. Faragon JJ, Piliero PJ. HAART drug interactions with recreational drugs. *AIDS Reader*, 2003, 13:433–450.

121. Harrington RD et al. Life-threatening interactions between HIV-1 protease inhibitors and the illicit drugs MDMA and gamma-hydroxybutyrate. *Archives of Internal Medicine*, 1999, 159:2221–2224.

122. Deeks SG. Determinants of virological response to antiretroviral therapy: implications for long-term strategies. *Clinical Infectious Diseases*, 2000, 30 (Suppl 2):S177–S184.

123. Wood E et al. Adherence to antiretroviral therapy and CD4 T-cell count responses among HIV-infected injection drug users. *Antiviral Therapy*, 2004, 9:229–235.

124. Bartlett JA. Addressing the challenges of adherence. *Journal of Acquired Immune Deficiency Syndromes*, 2002, 29:S2–S10.

125. Palepu A et al. Impaired virologic response to highly active antiretroviral therapy associated with ongoing injection drug use. *Journal of Acquired Immune Deficiency Syndromes*, 2003, 32:522–526.

126. Bangsberg DR et al. Adherence to protease inhibitors, HIV-1 viral load and development of drug resistance in an indigent population. *AIDS*, 2000, 14:357–366.

127. Bangsberg DR et al. High levels of adherence do not prevent the development of HIV antiretroviral drug resistance. *AIDS*, 2003, 17:1925–1932.

128. Singh N et al. Adherence of human immunodeficiency virus-infected patients to antiretroviral therapy. *Clinical Infectious Diseases*, 1999, 29:824–830.

129. Moatti JP et al. Adherence to HAART in French HIV-infected injecting drug users: the contribution of buprenorphine drug maintenance treatment. *Journal of Acquired Immune Deficiency Syndromes*, 2000, 14:151–155.

130. Wohl AR et al. A randomized trial of directly administered antiretroviral therapy and adherence case management intervention. *Clinical Infectious Diseases*, 2006, 42:1619–1627.

131. Wood E et. al. Rates of antiretroviral resistance among HIV-infected patients with and without a history of injection drug use. *AIDS*, 2005, 19:1189–1195.

132. Clarke S et al. Assessing limiting factors to the acceptance of antiretroviral therapy in a large cohort of injecting drug users. *HIV Medicine*, 2003, 4:33–37.

133. Wu C et al. Focus groups among intravenous drug users in Ruili, Yunnan province, China, to develop interventions to improve adherence to antiretrovirals. Presented at the XVI International AIDS Conference, Toronto, Canada, 13–18 August 2006. Abstract CDB0828.

134. Ickovics JR et al. Mortality, CD4 cell count decline, and depressive symptoms among HIV-seropositive women: longitudinal analysis from the HIV Epidemiology Research Study. *Journal of the American Medical Association*, 2001, 285:1466–1474.

135. Cruess DG et al. Association of depression, CD8+ T lymphocytes, and natural killer cell activity: implications for morbidity and mortality in human immunodeficiency virus disease. *Current Psychiatry Reports*, 2003(a), 5:445–450.

136. Ammassari A et al. Self reported symptoms and side-effects influence adherence to highly active antiretroviral therapy in persons with HIV infection. *Journal of Acquired Immune Deficiency Syndromes*, 2001, 28:445–449.

137. Spire B et al. Adherence to highly active antiretroviral therapies (HAART) in HIV-infected patients: from a predictive to a dynamic approach. *Social Science and Medicine*, 2002, 54:1481–1496.

138. Ware NC, Wyatt MA, Tugenberg T. Adherence, stereotyping and unequal HIV treatment for active users of illegal drugs. *Social Science and Medicine*, 2005, 61:565–576.

139. Carrieri MP et al. Impact of early versus late adherence to highly active antiretroviral therapy on immuno-virological response: a 3-year follow-up study. *Antiviral Therapy*, 2003(a), 8:585–594.

140. Safren SA et al. Two strategies to increase adherence to HIV antiretroviral medication: life steps and medication monitoring. *Behaviour Research and Therapy*, 2001, 39:1481–1496.

141. Simoni JM et al. Antiretroviral adherence interventions: a review of current literature and ongoing studies. *Topics in HIV Medicine*, 2003, 11:185–198.

142. Golin CE et al. Adherence counseling practices of generalist and specialist physicians caring for people living with HIV/AIDS in North Carolina. *Journal of General Internal Medicine*, 2004, 19:16–27.

143. Patrick D et al. Incidence of hepatitis C virus among drug users during an outbreak of HIV infection. *Canadian Medical Association Journal*, 2001, 165:889–895.

144. Smyth BP, Keenan E, O'Connor JJ. Blood borne viral infection in Irish injecting drug users. *Addiction*, 1998, 93:1649–1656.

145. Garten RJ et al. Rapid transmission of hepatitis C among young injecting heroin users in Southern China. *International Journal of Epidemiology*, 2004, 33:182–188.

146. Keating S et al. Hepatitis C viral clearance in an intravenous drug-using cohort in the Dublin area. *Irish Journal of Medical Science*, 2005, 174:37–41.

147. Grebely J et al. Hepatitis C virus reinfection in injection drug users. *Hepatology*, 2006, 44:1139–1145.

148. Renault PF et al. Psychiatric complications of long-term interferon-alpha therapy. *Archives of Internal Medicine*, 1987, 147:1577–1580.

149. Torriani FJ et al. Peginterferon alfa-2a plus ribavarin for chronic hepatitis C virus infection in HIV-infected patients. *New England Journal of Medicine*, 2004, 351:438–450.

150. Carrat F et al. Pegylated interferon alfa-2b vs. standard interferon alfa-2a plus ribavarin for chronic hepatitis C in HIV-infected patients: a randomized controlled trial. *Journal of the American Medical Association*, 2004, 292:2839–2848.

151. Chung R et al. Peginterferon alfa-2a plus ribavarin versus interferon alfa-2a plus ribavarin for chronic hepatitis C in HIV-co-infected patients. *New England Journal of Medicine*, 2004, 351:451–459.

152. Hung CC et al. Improved outcome of HIV-1 infected adults with tuberculosis in the era of highly active antiretroviral therapy. *AIDS*, 2003, 17:2615–2622.

153. Narita M et al. Use of rifabutin with protease inhibitors for HIV-infected patients with tuberculosis. *Clinical Infectious Diseases*, 2000, 30:779–783.

154. Rimland D et al. Prospective study of etiologic agent of community-acquired pneumonia in patients with HIV infection. *AIDS*, 2002, 16:85–95.